calm to chaos

calm to chaos

GARTH WADE

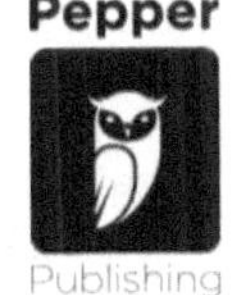

Pepper Publishing

PEPPER PUBLISHING
AUSTRALIA

Copyright © Garth Wade 2016

www.garthwade.com.au

A CIP catalogue reference for this book is available from the National Library of Australia.

Paperback ISBN 978-0-9953754-0-6
eBook ISBN 978-0-9953754-1-3

Printed and bound by IngramSpark/Lightning Source
eBook by KDP

calm to chaos /Garth Wade - 2nd ed.

Come back. Even as a shadow, even as a dream.
—Euripides

CONTENTS

Abbreviations

ACP – advanced care paramedic
ALOC – altered level of consciousness
APO – acute pulmonary oedema
BVM – bag valve mask
c-spine – cervical spine
CPAP – continuous positive airway pressure
CPR – cardiopulmonary resuscitation
CT – computed tomography
ED – emergency department
ECG – electrocardiogram
GTN – Glycerol Trinitrate
ICP – intensive care paramedic
MD/MDMA – methylenedioxymethamphetamine
OPA – oropharyngeal airway
PA – Princess Alexandra Hospital
PEA – pulseless electrical activity
QE2 – Queen Elizabeth II Jubilee Hospital
QFRS – Queensland Fire and Rescue Service
RTC – road traffic collision
SDU – Staff Development Unit
SITREP – a situation report
TIA – transient ischemic attack

18:55 hrs – Sydney

'It's like nothing you've ever felt before —'

'How do you know?' she said, wedging the phone into her shoulder and flipping through the book in her lap until she found her place – *Learn Spanish Rapido!*

'Because I know you, Amber, and you've never done anything that's even half as much fun.'

'Hey! I've done lots of fun things. Just because *you* don't think they're fun …'

'Okay, settle down, Ms Highly Strung.'

She gave a soft snort of amusement.

'All I'm saying is that it's a spectacular feeling. I'm sure you've had heaps of fun times in your life, but you can*not* have felt anything like this before.'

He heard her take a deep breath but he continued. 'Now hold on. I don't *care* that you don't like what I like. I don't mind that we have different hobbies. I think it's good to have some time away from each other occasionally, you know, so we're not living in each other's pockets. But I did really enjoy spending the whole day with you today …'

'So did I, even though we spent most of it in bed,' Amber said.

'Hey, you wanted to as much as I did,' he said, smiling.

'Well I wanted it more than I ever want to go skydiving, that's for sure.'

'I don't object to that at all my dear.'

'Don't call me "dear" Sydney – you sound like my grandpa.'

There was a pause, which Syd hurried to fill. 'So, how is the Spanish coming along? *Muy bien*?'

'The Spanish is coming along *very well* thank you. Just because you've travelled to Bolivia for *five* minutes!' She slipped the phone onto the sofa and put it on speaker. Syd's voice seemed more manageable when it wasn't in her ear.

'Okay, okay. But I've said I'll practise with you any time, hon, you know that. We'll be chatting *en Español* before you know it.'

Amber could hear how much he wanted to please her, to smooth over any awkwardness between them. She stretched her legs out along the sofa. She enjoyed staying over at Syd's townhouse, wedged into bayside Brisbane, the sky big and unhindered by tall buildings. This was one life path that she wanted to follow, to see where it led her. She watched the sky turn apricot as the sun sank towards the horizon, the light adding a warmth to her skin.

'And Amber, you really don't have to worry about me getting with the girls at the drop-zone, because I'm only interested in you ...'

She let the silence grow.

'... 'cause I love you.'

More silence. No reply at all. Just silence. He thought he could hear the network's digital stopwatch ticking over as it tallied up expensive seconds for the call.

Syd reminded himself of his motto – *Life is too short*.

Then she sighed. 'God, why do you have to get so ... serious all of a sudden? I ... love you too, you know ...'

Sydney let his breath go in a long exhalation. He could feel himself smiling, all the tightness in his eyes and cheeks.

Bee-beep – bee-beep.

'Hold on a sec,' she said, 'I've got another call.'

The silence over his phone became absolute. Syd kicked a stone and watched Cameron checking the ambulance and its supplies, being his usual responsible senior partner, making sure Syd hadn't missed anything. His face felt hot even though the warmth was fading from the sunlight. Syd remembered when, just two weeks ago, he'd said those three special little words to Amber. She'd hugged him and murmured something unintelligible, leaving Syd completely in the dark about how she felt.

Cameron leant in at the driver's side of the truck and fiddled with something. Syd heard a couple of beeps and realised Cam was probably logging on early. He didn't mind; he was keen. He heard a click over the phone, then her voice: 'Hey, I gotta go,' Amber said abruptly.

'Everything okay?'

'Oh … yeah … fine. Everything's fine. I'm, um, going round to Marcia's later. Gotta get ready.'

Syd felt the familiar vibration on his hip, then the shrill, constant beep of the pager.

LOGGED ON – PAGE – BRAVO 989 WELCOME TO NIGHT SHIFT—

'Are you working tonight?'

'Nah I've got two nights off. Hey, I've really gotta go,' Amber said.

Another vibration.

CODE 2A – 17B1 – FALL POSSIBLY DANGEROUS BODY AREA – WHITES HILL FOOTBALL FIELDS – CAMP HILL

'That's okay; I've got a job anyway.'

That familiar silence again. He thought he could hear her cogs turning.

'What kind of job?' she asked.

'I thought you had to go.'

'Just say, silly …'

'Just a fall. Won't know any more till I go inside to the truck.'

Another short silence – more cog turning. 'Where is it?'

'Why the interest all of a sudden?'

'I care about you, that's all.'

'Whites Hill … they'd be playing touch footy tonight I think.'

Silence. Awkward silence.

Syd broke it. 'So, I'll talk to you later tonight, yeah? Are you sure everything is okay?'

Amber paused. 'Um … yeah … I suppose … I'll talk to you later, okay? Yeah we really need to talk.'

Cameron mouthed something at Syd – 'We should go!'

'Okay then, chat later! *Adiós.*'

He jumped into the truck, turning his attention to the next job, the next patient. The details were on the screen, and Syd felt the familiar rush, the endorphins buzzing around his brain. It was like the first jump of the day, or that first time he sat packed in tightly with all the other skydivers, collectively knowing they would all soon fling themselves from the plane into thin icy air. Such exhilaration, such lusty, addictive energy, it was a rush that Syd found impossible to explain.

18:55 hrs – Sebastian

The grass was wet and cold, but he rarely felt the fresh crunch of frost underfoot here. Sebastian could see his breath in the light streaming from the towers at each corner of the field, and heat rose from the other men's shoulders and heads.

The Mustangs (Tuesday night A-Grade Men's Touch Football) had a catchphrase: 'Constant speed, forward movement and aggressive defence.' Sebastian thought it sounded silly. Sometimes, he would look in the mirror before a game and pretend a sports reporter was interviewing him. 'Yes I think it is important to be competitive but I don't like to, ah how do you say it … "rabbit on" with crazy slogans, I just like to play.' He thought of himself as a good-natured Latino man who didn't take life too seriously.

He was a team player, and a good one, but his teammates sensed he didn't much like the machismo, the blokey camaraderie and post-match boozing, and because of this he was always something of an outsider. Until, that is, the team was losing. Then, every one of the five other men on the field would try their damnedest to get the ball to Sebastian, knowing that almost every time he had it he would do well. And when that happened all was forgiven – high fives, hugs and bum-slaps all round.

Sebastian's side's green jerseys pushed forward, as the red team defended, bouncing backwards off their opposition signalling a touch. Green hands, pass, touch. Ball to ground. Green hands, pass, pass, touch, ball to ground. Speedy. Green team hands, ran across the field drawing the extra defender and leaving a gap as wide as a garage door. Sebastian was heading toward his touchdown zone. 'Yes,' he said, much too quietly for a football field, but loud enough for his teammate to hear. A backhanded flick pass seemed to float for a second before Sebastian soared forward, catching the ball against his flank and running like a gazelle.

The pass wrong-footed most of the other players, but one red-shirt remained, closing in on Sebastian from the right. As the red-shirt cut off his angle, Sebastian lengthened his stride and swerved to the left side of the field, eyes fixed in a sharp glare, thick black hair streaming behind him. He grasped the ball firmly in one large hand – he could almost hear his old coach screaming in fury – as his arms pumped like pistons, his shirt flattened against his lean, muscular torso. Despite the frosty air, he felt sweat sliding down his face.

He had one more opposition player to beat, and his teammates would never catch up. The gap between the two men had almost closed when, at the last second, Sebastian planted one foot hard on the ground and tried to sidestep his assailant. The power of that forward charge abruptly stopping shot through the bones of his left leg as it skewed to one side and snapped the fibula. All the kinetic energy was then transferred to the tibia, which broke jaggedly, pushing down towards the ankle, piercing the surrounding skin and muscle, retracting slightly as the calf muscle clenched. As both bones in his lower left leg fractured, Sebastian hit the ground. Hard. *Now* the grass felt crunchy.

He writhed in agony, screaming as the pain flared up his leg, grabbing uselessly at his perforated shin. He dragged in a ragged breath through his nostrils, trying to lie still. He pushed his head into the grass, shutting his eyes against the blinding floodlights as he wrestled with the pain. He opened his eyes as he heard the thud of approaching feet and saw his breath mist through the air.

'Oh shit. That really hurts.'

18:55 hrs – Cameron

Cam smoothed out Syd's letter on the dashboard and settled down to read.

To Whom It May Concern,

My name is Sydney Worthington and I moved from New South Wales nine months ago for this job.

I have chosen to write down some of the happenings in my life through last year, and how they may have affected me during the first stage of my learning as a student paramedic.

Firstly, I must state that I always had the opportunity to let the officers and assessors at the Staff Development Unit (SDU) know of these events, and when I did see those officers, for either assessments or learning-support plans, they always asked if I had any problems or issues in my personal life that might have been affecting my learning.

I always replied with a very definite 'No'. I answered in this way because I didn't want anyone to think I was making excuses for my failures in my studies. Now my job is on the line, so the time has come to inform this Review Panel of the factors that have been affecting me, to try to provide some insight and maybe clarification of my circumstances, rather than making excuses.

Late last year, my girlfriend and I broke up. I won't go into the details of it, but as most people know, a break-up, no matter how uncomplicated or unproblematic, is never an easy thing.

In mid-August, my mother, who lives in New South Wales, informed me she had recently been diagnosed with breast cancer. Not only was this a huge shock to her but also a shock for me, and an obvious ongoing concern. Over the next two months, even though my involvement in my mum's cancer treatment was limited, it definitely took a toll on my ability to concentrate and work. On top of that, at the beginning of September, she went into atrial fibrillation, and while it was managed quickly and effectively, the worry was definitely an added pressure for me.

Then, no less than a month later, my grandmother, who also lives in New South Wales, also went into atrial fibrillation for three days. My family has a history of good health, so having two family members' with health problems is a new concept for me, one I have naively never really thought about until now.

I have always been proactive towards learning in past jobs, wishing to become a better worker and to increase my understanding and productivity, and always approached learning with enthusiasm. However, most of the learning I have done in the past has been task orientated, and I haven't had my 'head in the books' since Year 12, which was almost ten years ago. Obviously I was not prepared for the study that is involved in the diploma. I was, and still am, absolutely committed, but I just didn't realise how much book-work was involved.

My girlfriend and I are back together. Our relationship is stable and our bond is strong.

My mother had radiation therapy, which destroyed the cancer. She is now on Femara and Aspirin.

My grandmother's sweet heart has now returned to a normal sinus rhythm. She continues to make nice biscuits.

I appreciate that I will always face challenges. Everybody has challenges and factors that affect their life. I would like to ask for your understanding about why I lacked focus last year. Now that I have seen the level of book-work that is involved, and have been told repeatedly that it will increase in volume and complexity throughout the diploma, I have gained a new focus, one that I hope I will have the opportunity to make routine.

I love working for this service. I love this job. I have never done a job where I get back so much from helping people. I love speaking with new people and going to different places. I find the high times exciting and the slow times give room to study and learn.

I love being on-road. I love being involved and making myself useful in situations ranging from a simple lift-assist, to a cyanosed APO, to extricating patients in an RTC.

Do I have a learning difficulty? No. I have to *practise* more scenarios, get the systems completely automated in my head, and allocate more time before assessments. *I have to study, I have to write notes, I have to get my 'head in the books', and I absolutely have to establish a routine.* I didn't really even know how to do that before, but after certain service people gave me some help, I now know my learning style and what I need to do to make the information stick.

I can do well at this job. I can learn to be a good paramedic. Please know that I will do what I need to do to make it happen.

Thank you.

Regards,

Sydney Worthington.

19:01 hrs – Bravo Unit 989

'Well your letter sounds like a right load of shite then, doesn't it?' Cam said in his thick Scots accent.

'Yeah, thanks for your support Cam. Your feedback could be a little bit more constructive though, mentor!'

'Yeah I know. I'm havin' a go. I think it's pretty bloody well written for someone like you!'

'Again, thanks,' Syd grinned, 'dick.' He concentrated on typing job details onto the iPad on his lap as they drove to the job at the sports field.

'I reckon you'll be all right, you'll probably just get a rousin' on for tellin' that supervisor off.' Cam grinned. 'Actually, they might fire you just for that!'

Sydney found himself having to concentrate whenever Cameron spoke, his words often obscured by his accent.

'I knew you were going to bring that up. I haven't written about it because they know who was at fault – their inept staff member at the SDU! That matter is settled. And I'd like them to try and fire me for that, or to even make mention of it actually. I'll quickly put on my lawyer hat for that. I'd be David, they'd be Goliath. I'd love to take on a big government company and teach them a lesson. Like Erin Brockovich. Ooh yes, Julia Roberts is so hot in that!'

Cameron concentrated on his driving. He always drove the ambulance at exactly the speed limit. The traffic built up behind them.

'So you're a lawyer now?' Cam said, when the road cleared ahead of them. 'I doubt that, Sydney. You're having trouble getting past assessment one point one, let alone being able to take an ambulance service to court and represent yourself! Fookin' crazy man! And what's this biblical reference? I thought you hated religion.' Cam drove with one hand on the wheel, in a constant state of awareness.

'Well, maybe I'll just get a good lawyer instead. And we're not getting into a discussion on religion again – you couldn't handle the last one we had.' Syd looked over at Cameron and added with steely determination, 'I am going to pass this next assessment you know.'

'I know you will, son. You just gotta learn how to play the game. Since I've been with you, we've worked well together, and you're more on the ball than you need to be on most jobs. I've got nothin' but praise for you, lad. You just gotta learn the exam and scenario stuff and all will be well.'

'I know. And I will. Like I said in the letter, which I am reading *out loud* to the head honchos next week.'

'Oh oh oh, that'll be a good one, 'cause you've answered everything in the letter that those idiots will ask, and they'll be stuck for questions. You watch them. Mate, they'll just look confused and then get out the novelty-sized bahookie smacker and redden your cheeks for you!' Cam smirked as he pictured Syd bent over a desk yelping as one of the overweight 'teachers' from the SDU spanked his behind.

As the ambulance eventually neared the sports field, Cameron turned off the main road onto a dirt track and followed it up an embankment toward a vast expanse of playing fields. The bright colours of the many different team uniforms ran back and forth on each field, looking busy and frenzied, and which lit up like a carnival.

'Oh, there we go. Yes, mate, I can see you … you're definitely wavin'. You're not drownin' …' Cam said, as he locked eyes on the 'waver', who clearly wanted to ensure Cam and Syd saw him, even though they were now only thirty metres away and had an unobstructed view of the whole scene. They crossed one field and drove onto another, the ambulance coming to a halt beside a dark-skinned man in a green sports shirt who had been laid on his back and covered by a blanket. Three worried onlookers in the same shirts surrounded him.

Syd jumped out of the passenger side and was met by another man wearing a red sports shirt.

'Hi there, how are you doing?'

'Well thanks, you?' Syd tried not to be abrupt.

'Well, I'm okay, but my mate on the opposition here isn't doing too well. I'm Tim, a doctor at the QE2.' Tim motioned towards the man on the ground. 'This is Sebastian, a twenty-six year old male with no medical history, allergies nor medications. Tonight he was witnessed attempting to sidestep another player, falling over, and sustaining a severe injury to his left lower leg. On examination he has deformity to his left ankle. I don't have any drugs here, so he's had no pain relief, and we haven't moved him from where he fell. He says he can still feel his toes but I haven't seen them.'

Syd raised an eyebrow and said, 'Wow, that's possibly the best handover I've ever had. Thank you very much.' He smiled, turned away from Tim and knelt down to the left of his patient. 'Hi there, what's your name?'

The felled man spoke through the fog of pain in a thick Latino accent. 'Ah … my name … is … Sebastian.'

'Okay, Sebastian, my name's Sydney and that's Cameron over there. Our friendly doctor on the opposition team tells me you've done some damage to your lower left leg, yes? Can you point to it and tell me if ten was the worst pain you've ever had in your life and zero was nothing, what number would you give you pain now?' Syd gently pressed Sebastian's inner wrist, intuitively counting a pulse rate.

'The pain I feel, it is … very bad.'

'Cam, can you get the Methoxy happening, vitals, then set up for cannulation please.'

'No problem.'

'Sebastian, we are going to take care of this pain, this leg, and you, and get you off to hospital okay? What I need you to do is just *try* to relax. I know it's not the easiest thing right now, but if you can just concentrate on your breathing … nice … and slow … and steady …' Syd demonstrated what he wanted his patient to do, '… and while you're busy relaxing, I'm going to have a look at you and ask some more questions, and Cameron's going to get you something for the pain, okay?'

'Mmm, okay, yes,' groaned Sebastian.

'Now, have you got any problems with your liver

or kidneys?'

'No.'

'And have you ever heard of something called malignant hyperthermia?'

'No.'

'Have you got any allergies?'

'No.'

'And what is your medical history?'

'My what?'

'Have you got any medical conditions or been to hospital or seen a doctor recently?'

'Ah. No. But I broke my wrist ... when I was a kid. That is it.'

'Great, well Cam's going to give you a thing like a whistle that you can breathe on for pain relief. Have you ever had a cigarette before?'

'Yes, and I didn't like it.'

'Well this is used in the same way; just breathe it in gently to start because it might make you cough. Then afterwards you'll hopefully get some relief from it. If you cover up that little hole on the top it'll give you a bigger hit.' Cameron handed Sydney a green whistle and a small empty bottle. Syd quickly inspected the bottle, read out the drug name and expiry date and handed the whistle to his patient. 'Just remember to go easy to start with ... you understand what I'm saying? Yes?'

'Yes ... I understand.'

Syd released Sebastian's wrist and moved up to

his head, where he put a hand each side and said, 'Sebastian, just keep on with that whistle, but can you tell me if you got knocked out in the fall?'

'No, I did not.'

'So you remember the whole thing?'

'Yes.'

'Have you got any neck pain at all?'

'No.'

'Did you hit your head on another player's knee or anything crazy like that?'

'No.'

Syd turned towards Cam. 'You happy with that? No ALOC. Does have distracting injuries but I don't think the mechanism is enough for c-spine concerns.'

'Yep. Just take it easy on that foot before you rip that boot off … we'll get his pain under control first, yeah?' Cameron said, monitoring Syd's actions.

'For sure. Now, Sebastian, while you're taking some nice big puffs on that whistle, Cam is going to give you a needle in your hand so we can give you some stronger pain relief,' said Syd.

'The good stuff?' Sebastian's accent was endearing.

'Hey, how do you know about the good stuff? But yep that's right, the good stuff!' Syd grinned as he quickly moved down to Sebastian's blanketed feet.

'I am from South America, man, we *invented* the

good stuff!' he said, still squinting.

His legs were splayed, turned out at the knees, but with both football booted feet pointing to the right at the same angle. Heat radiated from his dark, solid thighs.

Syd gently held Sebastian's booted left foot at the toes and at the heel. 'Hey Sebastian, is this the sore leg?' he said kindly, not trying to be comical.

'Yes,' Sebastian said, his attention taken by the other paramedic who finished wrapping the blood-pressure cuff around his arm. 'But hold on … what is this guy doing to me again?'

Cam then tightened a tourniquet around Sebastian's forearm, and said in his booming friendly voice, 'I'm gonna put a wee needle in your hand so we can make this leg feel better … remember? The gooood stuff?'

'Okay, I will relax,' Sebastian replied. Cam found the vein promptly on the healthy young arm and quickly inserted the needle. He then read the drug out loud and showed it to Syd before drawing it up and administering it via the green plastic tube protruding from Sebastian's right hand, fixed with a neat plaster.

'Excellent!' Syd directed his voice down the length of his patient's body. 'Remember that zero to ten scale? Now what number is that pain you've got in your leg?'

'I think about an eight.'

'Okay my friend, for now just keep sucking on that whistle. We'll give that Morphine a couple of minutes to work before I take this boot off …'

The games on the other fields continued, and Syd heard distant cries of 'Yes!', 'Slide!', 'No!', Slide across!'. People were running, leaping, yelling. Syd found it distracting – he knew the game well, and had been playing for a number of years. As the minutes passed he found himself wanting to watch.

'Hey Sebastian, how are you feeling up there?'

'Hey man … I feel okay …' he said casually.

'What number is that pain, amigo?'

'Oh, it is about at a two.'

'Well, I'm going to take this boot off your foot now. I will go slowly and gently, so just tell me if it hurts too much, okay?'

'Yes, I will tell you man.'

Syd had already undone the laces and cut down the length of the sock against the ankle. The deformity was obvious – the sock bulged where the foot entered the boot. After carefully manoeuvring the boot without a word from the patient, Syd eased it off, and cut the sock away completely. He was relieved to see a sweaty left foot with good colour and warm to the touch. Around two centimetres of glistening white bone protruded through the skin and rested against the top of the foot. There was no blood. Syd could feel a strong, regular pedal pulse.

'So, Sebastian, what I want you to do is just stay

nicely relaxed and continue not to move your leg or foot. You've fractured one, maybe both of the bones in your lower leg, so we're going to clean it, wrap it and deliver you nicely to hospital where they might operate. We're also going to look after the pain you feel and make sure that all-important blood keeps making its way to your toes.'

'I don't remember all of what you just said, but thank you, you guys are fantastico!' said the groggy footballer.

'Can you feel me doing this?' Syd gently pinched each of Sebastian's toes, noting how quickly the colour returned after each pinch and checking for affirmation each time. 'And … what number is that pain now?' Syd's tone had shifted to mild-mannered game-show host, but not too flashy and without the cheesy grin. Asking the same question repeatedly was boring – he liked to spice it up a little.

'It is coming back … a little …' Sebastian replied.

'Can you give another five please, Cam.' Syd was busy at the man's feet, supporting the injury and rinsing blades of grass from the bone, which had strangely appeared despite being protected by the sock.

'Sure about another five?' Cam said, testing.

'With his size, his age, the injury sustained and the fact we are going to have to move his leg, I am absolutely sure.'

Cam had already started to deliver some more of

the good stuff through Sebastian's cannula. Soon after, he joined Syd and helped to raise Sebastian's leg slightly and vacuum-splint the injury. Some of Sebastian's teammates helped lift him onto the scoop stretcher before he was transferred to the ambulance stretcher then into the vehicle.

Cameron checked that all was well with his partner and his patient before slamming the sliding cabin door shut and slowly driving off the field.

19:30 hrs – Amber

She entered his empty apartment just as she did on any other day, cruising on in to the beeping of the security system. She tapped in the security code, placed the key on the crafted hall table and walked through to the mildly opulent bedroom to gather some clothes and toiletries for him.

She liked to think she was always cool, and was never stirred up, and never got angry or over-emotional. She was rarely upset, and most certainly never in the presence of another person.

She hurried, but she never rushed. Above all, she always, always got her own way.

19:30 hrs – Club Outlook Park, Morningside

Bradley and Ken met at the usual place in run-of-the-mill suburbia, a children's park with a golf course on one side and a small artificial lake on the other. The surrounding houses, each of which was one of ten different architectural 'masterpieces', had slightly different coloured bricks, or shaded guttering, or rose bushes, but there were no leaves on the ground and no mess. Brand-spanking-new suburbia.

Ken read some of the surrounding signs: 'Planned perfection!' 'Exceptional investment opportunity!' 'Second to none!' 'Stunning showcase display village!' 'Land, location, luxury!' *Live more.*

Now. Yours for only $349,000!'

All of the houses had been packed in so closely around the narrow courts and roads that swinging a cat in the front yards would be a mean feat. Clearly the $349,000 didn't include any privacy. But living here seemed to make people happy. And normal, he supposed.

Ken stood near a rare tree beside a mini swing set. He was wearing a green tracksuit that, like the suburb, appeared brand new.

Bradley approached him across the park with a ridiculous self-assurance, strutting in a way that Ken had initially put down to some sort of leg injury.

Ken cleared his throat, his breath condensing in the night air – unusual for this time of year. Bradley, whose clothing was not so new and not so fresh, studied Ken for a moment then said, 'What's up, mate?'

Ken pushed his round glasses up the bridge of his nose, 'Nothing, Brad, nothing, but I'd prefer to make this quick if we can. I'm really sorry, but there's been a change of—'

'Hang on man, you sayin' a change? A change of plans? So, you *tell* me what you want, which I have *with* me, then I show up at the *time, date and place* we have established for this meeting … and you have a *change of plans*? Shit man, this'll wanna work out for me …' Bradley's accent was straight out of Los Angeles gangland, although he had never travelled beyond his home state in Australia. Clearly, he'd been catching up on the genre.

'Of course it will, Brad. Like I said, I'm very sorry. It's just that I need *more*, and I was hoping you'd have more with you ...' Ken said gingerly, 'but I don't suppose you have?'

'Now why would I bring more than the required amount? *Think*, man!' Bradley seemed jumpy.

'I'm terribly sorry, but I have only just been informed of my party's change of plans,' Ken said.

Bradley sighed ostentatiously. 'So, how much you need?'

'Twenty ecstasy, twenty coke, ten rohypnol, if that's okay?'

'I ain't got near that on me, man.' Bradley glanced around the dimly lit park, 'but we can meet back here in an hour, yeah?'

'Okay then. Sorry again to call you out and change the order. It was all just very last minute.'

'Hey, no problemo. My customers ask, and I provide.' Bradley held up his arms like a bishop. 'And it'll be seven K too. That's good clean coke and those E's that you like from last time.'

'Jesus! Seven grand?' Ken bit his lip, knowing he was cornered. He shifted his weight. 'Oh well, okay, don't suppose we really have any other options.'

'No doubt you don't,' Bradley was confident in his grammar and even sounded cocky now, 'and you know what; I'll throw the roofies in for free.'

'Hardly free for seven grand,' muttered Ken, 'but thanks.'

'See you back here in an hour exactly.'

*

Lorraine peered across the golf course. Although it was night, she could clearly see the telltale stripes of The Idiot's tracksuit as he got out of his car and walked into a children's park. She referred to Bradley as The Idiot whenever he proved to her that he would always be a no-hoper, which was regularly, due to his replicating behaviour.

She knew he'd lied to her – predictable as a losing lottery ticket.

As she watched the two figures talking, she felt the buzz. Her heart rate increased, her skin goose-pimpled, and she felt the need for a deep steadying breath. She loved this feeling. She knew it was an addiction.

She jumped into her car and sped back to Bradley's house in Carina. Sweat slicked her palms as she gripped the steering wheel hard. She wound down the window and felt the breeze cooling her face and neck. She felt exhilarated. She knew there would be more of this excitement soon, very soon. She raced around each corner, loving the swoop of the car, listening to the tyres screech, but she slowed to less than the speed limit as she approached her destination.

Bradley's house was a single-storey, multi-coloured brick and fibro-cement home with metal roofing. It was impossible to tell whether the fibro or brick had come first, but it was one of the ugliest houses in the whole suburb. The front yard was dirt and gravel from the house to the unpainted picket fence, and the nature strip was much the same, apart from the occasional patch of dying grass: a typical poverty-ridden, housing-commission shit-heap.

She stroked the keys between her thumb and forefinger, wondering if she should go in. She knew intellectually that what she intended to do was 'wrong' – it would have a hugely detrimental effect on Bradley's life, but not really on anybody else's – and really, she would be doing the community a service. Besides, the thrill was addictive. She was hooked.

She thought of what her father would say, and felt her heart clench.

Leaping out of her car, she shut the door quietly and, being sure not to appear to sneak, entered Bradley's house using the key he had entrusted to her. The interior had been quite nicely renovated, in contrast to the houso exterior. The painting complemented the entrance tiles nicely, the lounge room was comfortable and clean, and there were quality fittings and carpets throughout. Someone with a good eye for design had influenced the interior furnishing decisions.

Lorraine checked every room, making sure Bradley hadn't somehow beaten her back, heard her, and was perhaps hiding for a joke. He wasn't, so she re-entered the main bedroom, scanned the room quickly then produced a key from her hip pocket that she had had cut months ago, predicting that a night like this would eventually come.

She carefully opened the sliding wardrobe door, knelt down and looked intently at the shoes on the bottom shelf. She shifted them to the left with professional care. Her hands were smooth and sure as she moved to the safe, her breathing flat and composed.

The key creaked in the lock, followed a second later by the click of the retracting bolt. Lorraine leant to one side so the dull streetlight could shine into the safe; it was just enough for her to make out the contents.

She grabbed the small rectangular box and stood up. She felt calm but alert, as though she had done this a million times before, ready to take flight if need be.

There was not a sound in the house.

She opened the rectangular black box and saw two hypodermic syringes still in their packaging. She tipped the lot into her hand: two alcohol swabs, a stick of filter, a small plastic baggie of heroin, and two round, green OxyContin tablets.

Lorraine fished out a replica of Bradley's baggie, and switched the two, replacing everything in the black box, then she shut it all up carefully, and placed it back in the safe. She slid the key into the lock and listened to the bolt slide into place. She took her time replacing the shoes: one lace in one lace out on the left shoe, angled at forty-five degrees to the right, which snuggled up flat next to the other.

Her knees cracked as she stood. She caught a sharp trace of Bradley's deodorant and quickly turned her head, her heart rate rising. Nobody was there.

She settled, blew a kiss into the wardrobe, and slid shut the door.

19:35 hrs – Bravo Unit 989

'How are you feeling, Sebastian?' Syd asked.

'Aw, man, I feel okay, it does not hurt like it was before, you know?'

'Well that's excellent news. I just want you to tell me if anything changes, yes? A new pain? Or a numb feeling at all in that leg or foot? You let me know straight away, okay?'

'Yes, I will tell you … aah I am sorry, I have forgotten your name …'

'I'm Sydney, and that's Cameron up front. Now, can you feel me touching your toes?'

'Yes.'

'And here?' Sydney circled his pen on Sebastian's heel, which he could only just reach at the end of the vacuum splint.

'Yes.'

'Can you wiggle your toes? Just a little bit.'

Sebastian concentrated, gripped the railing of the stretcher, and wiggled all the toes on the injured leg, ever so slightly. Sydney again noted the good colour and temperature of his patient's foot, then sat back in the chair, looking through the cab and windscreen, trying to work out their location.

'Excuse me driver, how far away are we?' Syd said, while trying to catch Cam's eye in the rear-view mirror.

'About five minutes, bearer,' Cam answered without taking his eyes off the road. 'Everything okay?'

'Everything's good,' Syd said, then turned his attention again to Sebastian. 'So, Sebastian, where are you from? How long have you been in Australia?' He was genuinely interested, and not just looking for a way to pass the time.

'I have been here for nine months and I came here for my job in Argentina,' Sebastian said comfortably.

'Oh man, that's great! I just got back from Bolivia – well a few months ago now – but I travelled over there at the end of last year. Man I loved it; I backpacked from La Paz to the jungle and back, it was so much fun! Have you been to Bolivia?' There were certain subjects, travel included, that got Syd instantly enthused. His family's favourite tease was to wonder aloud if there was some way to bottle his excitement and monopolise the energy drink market.

'No, I have not been to Bolivia, it doesn't interest me you know? But Argentina ... sí ... now this is a beautiful place.'

'Aah man, it's right next door to your country, and so many great places and people and the jungle and deserts and cities there are like nothing in Australia. Don't get me wrong, I love Australia, but South America is like another world! Do you miss home? Are you from Buenos Aires? I didn't go there but I can't wait to go again. I'll definitely go to Argentina!'

'Sí, I am from Buenos Aires, but it is just my home you know? I don't really think about that stuff ... just like you maybe don't think about kangaroos and Arse Rock to be that fun or exciting, you know?'

Syd smiled. He was enjoying the Latin accent, the strange pronunciations.

'You are laughing at my voice, huh?' Sebastian said, also smiling.

'Not your voice, your accent,' Syd said with a quiet chuckle. 'I'm sure the ladies love it.'

'Sí sí sí! Yes, some do for sure!' Sebastian's words sounded slightly slurred but he was still full of pep. 'But,' he looked down at his injured leg, 'I have a girlfriend, and she don't like it when I talk to other girls.'

'So you can only talk to blokes? Jeez that gets a bit boring after a while doesn't it?'

'Ah, nah I talk to girls, but just not too much, and not around my girlfriend, you understand?'

Cameron's voice echoed through the ambulance, 'Sorry guys, the road is terrible here, it'll be bumpy for a bit.'

'Thanks Cam,' Sydney said. Most roads around Brisbane were good and reasonably smooth, but bottoming out in one of the many small-child-sized potholes was still a regular occurrence. Cam had a reputation for driving like a Sunday afternoon retiree when patients were onboard the ambulance, something that occasionally annoyed the much less experienced and consequently more impatient Sydney.

'How's your pain Sebastian?' Syd asked as the vehicle began to rock.

'Ah, yes, I can feel the pain coming back very much now,' Sebastian said.

Syd checked his patient's blood pressure, which had been automatically taken forty-five seconds ago, and after confirming with Cam, administered further anaesthesia then flushed it through.

'I dunno Sebastian,' said Syd, bracing himself between the stretcher and the fridge, 'do you reckon it's a good thing she's so envious about simple things like you talking to other girls?'

Sebastian looked up at Syd, momentarily distracted from his splinted leg. 'Yes, my friend, I know what you mean, but,' Sebastian's eyes widened, 'she's got her secrets, and I got mine!' The Latin lover shot a wry smile at Syd.

'Ah, I see. I know what you're saying.' Syd paused, juggling the Morphine and flush syringes. 'I used to go out with a woman who would say, "If you spot it; you've got it"'.

Sebastian looked completely nonplussed. 'I am sorry Sydney, you are speaking a little too quickly. I do not understand what you are saying.'

'That's okay, mate. I didn't understand what she meant either at first, but eventually she explained.' Syd slowed his speech. 'She meant that if one person in a relationship is worried or paranoid about a certain behaviour in the other person, then it is probably that first person who is behaving that way. You understand?'

Sebastian still looked confused.

Syd explained. 'It's like your girlfriend always worrying you're going to cheat on her with another woman. It probably means she'd like to cheat on you with another guy.' He looked at his Latino patient to make sure he understood then added hastily, 'but that's not necessarily true. I'm just saying what she said. In fact, it's actually quite stupid now that I've said it out loud.'

'So, you are saying that you think maybe my

girlfriend talks to lots of other men? And that is suspicious? That maybe she's doing other things too?'

'No, no, I don't want to make any assumptions or judgements, particularly of someone I don't know anything about.' Syd paused. 'I'm just saying, my ex-girlfriend, well, a woman I dated, used to believe this. It's not necessarily what I believe. Don't worry about it, Sebastian, it really is absolutely ridiculous.'

19:39 hrs – 47 Summer Street, Coorparoo

Ken's house was one of the more pretentious ones, with a ludicrously-sized fountain between the house and the driveway, and a thick rounded hedge separating the front garden from the street.

Bradley had slipped down the driveway of a house in Summer Street. It was all in darkness and gave him a good view of Ken's house. He caught sight of Ken walking over the large Italian harlequin porch tiles before he tapped on the front door of his house.

Ken's wife opened the door – a thin, pretty woman with a blonde bob – kissed him on the lips and smiled as he walked in.

The white stripes of Bradley's dark tracksuit gleamed in the streetlights as he slipped from house to house.

He crept towards Ken's house and crouched alongside the thick hedge by the driver's side of Ken's car. He squatted there for forty-five minutes, in which time he considered his options. Despite a total inability to change some harmful elements in his own life, Bradley always liked to consider his alternatives.

He thought *maybe* he could walk back around the corner to his car, drive home, and just not go through with the deal. That way he would only have *kind of* broken his promise to Lorraine. Or, he could *maybe* drive back to his house, get the drugs that Ken wanted, and meet him back at the park, as planned, to complete an 'honest' deal, but that would mean *completely* breaking his promise to Lorraine. Or *maybe* he could follow up on the idea that had slowly surfaced in his mind: if he put on his balaclava and mugged Ken of the $7000, thus only *partially* breaking his promise to Lorraine, he'd end up with free money *and* his drugs.

He settled on the latter, as he knew he would, and continued to watch, squatting like a Vietnamese farmer. After all, he was giving up the dealing, gradually, and this would definitely be a step in the right direction, although he failed to see the irony of keeping the drugs himself.

All at once Bradley doubted his decision. What if Ken had to go somewhere else to get the money, and would be coming out of his house with nothing close to the $7000 he was after? He pondered this for a moment, unable to think of a way he could ensure the money would be there when he reached for it. Then suddenly he heard movement inside the house, a loud laugh then muffled words before the front door opened, closed, and then footsteps crunched on the gravel driveway. Bradley felt a jet of adrenaline, and instinctively looked through the side windows of the car to confirm who was approaching. It was Ken.

Ken hurried past the front of his car, and Bradley heard his own knees click loudly as he propelled himself up and forward, grabbed Ken by the scruff of the shirt and forced him down onto the gravel between the car and the hedge. Bradley punched him hard on the nose and Ken let out a pained grunt. As balaclava-clad Bradley set about searching through the jacket of his punch-shocked client, Ken fumbled for the tiny handheld stun gun in the pocket of his pants. Bradley found the rolled-up wad of money in the inside front pocket of the jacket, grabbed it and squeezed it in his hand.

Ken struggled, slipped out of Bradley's grasp and scuttled sideways. Bradley lost his balance and found himself on both knees, then somehow pitching backwards. Ken felt a sudden surge of courage, spat out the blood filling his mouth, sat up and pushed the mugger backwards and onto his behind. He still couldn't find the stun gun, fumbling through his deep pockets as he struggled to his feet.

In a submissive and vulnerable posture that felt dangerously unfamiliar, Bradley saw Ken searching for something. He pulled up the leg of his own tracksuit pants and reached for his leg holster, extricating a small, clean knife.

In the same instant, Ken found the stun gun and stood over Bradley, holding it out in front of him as he'd seen men do in movies. Bradley held the knife towards Ken – he'd seen the same movies. There was a moment's standoff, then Bradley lunged at Ken and pushed the point of the knife to his chest then quickly withdrew it.

Ken, red with anger and buoyed on a surge of rage and power he never realised he possessed, pressed the stun gun hard against Bradley's stomach, with no effect whatsoever. He pushed the button as hard as he could and pressed the gun onto Bradley's chest, listening to the nasty, clattering sound it made – still nothing.

Bradley had fallen back again, grazing his knuckles clutching the money on the gravel. He watched as Ken dropped the stun gun, clutched at his chest, then turned and hurried back to the verandah. 'Help,' he said quietly, almost politely.

Bradley gripped his knife, grabbed Ken's stun gun and the money and ran. He was scratching at his chest and stomach by the time he reached his car. He threw himself into the seat and drove away, parking his car in an inconspicuous area surrounded by trees, not far from his house. He closed his eyes and slept.

19:55 hrs – Princess Alexandra Hospital Emergency Department

The ambulance reversed up to the ED, where five other ambulances were already parked. Syd thought it couldn't be a very busy night, but even if it had been, he knew they'd scoot through triage because he'd phoned through earlier. Sebastian was expected.

Cam gently rolled the stretcher carrying Sebastian into the ED and past Syd, who stopped to speak with the triage nurse. The hospital seemed quiet and the staff behind the counter were relaxed, both of which were rarely seen. There were no other patients in the resus beds so the triage nurse was happy for the newly arrived patient to go straight through, where a consultant, his trainee graduate doctor, and three other nurses were waiting.

They all looked at Syd as a nurse asked, 'Is this the compound tib-fib?'

Syd replied confidently, 'Sure is. If you'd like to give us a hand to get him over, then I'll hand over. Or I can do the two things at once, whichever you like.'

'There's no rush is there? Still no altered perfusion to that foot?' the nurse asked.

'Nothing's changed,' Syd replied, then told Sebastian that they were going to put a hard board under his back and slide him from the stretcher to the hospital bed. Sebastian seemed comfortable and followed instructions, keeping still and letting the medical staff do all the work.

'So, this is Sebastian, a twenty-six-year-old who was playing touch football, had a fall while running, and sustained a compound fracture to the lower left leg at around seven o'clock tonight. As you'll see, he has about two centimetres of exposed bone, with nil altered sensation, colour or temperature and with good movement to all toes. He has kept a sweet and steady pedal pulse and had a similar posterior tibial pulse before we vacuum splinted. At no time was there altered level of consciousness, patient remembers the whole event, and although the mechanism was enough to produce a compound fracture, there was reportedly never any impact with another player or object. Nil neck pain or tenderness. Pain has been managed with 3 ml Methoxyflurane, 12.5 mg Morphine plus 10 mg Metaclopromide, with vitals remaining within normal limits. Patient has no allergies and no history of lower leg fractures nor issues. Any questions?'

The resus team listened attentively to Syd's handover while examining, prodding and assessing Sebastian. Doctor Deepak Das, a consultant with a reputation for straight talking and for producing the best orthopaedic surgeons on the east coast, was about to speak when he was interrupted by a fiery-haired intern. 'What measures have been taken to ensure left-sided distal perfusion for this patient?' he asked in a nasal voice. The young man was overdressed in a brand-name French-cuffed shirt, trousers and dress shoes, an outfit that was just asking to be vomited on in the ED.

Syd looked at the intern, then at the consultant, and delicately raised a quizzical eyebrow. He had handed over to Doctor Das a number of times before and felt they had developed a professional rapport. He drew in a breath but Doctor Das cut him off, looking sharply at the intern and saying, 'Quiet.'

He turned back to Syd and said, 'Thank you Syd and to you also Cameron.' He gestured behind Syd to Cam, who was sheeting the cleaned stretcher.

'Not a worry Doc,' said the tall Scotsman.

'Excellent. 3 Methoxy, 12.5 Morph, and 10 Max. We'll have this vac splint at triage after we x-ray and decide on a plan.'

'No probs Doc. Good luck,' Syd finally turned to Sebastian, 'and good luck to you *amigo. Adiós.*'

'*Gracias amigo.* "If they spot it, they got it!"' he replied, smiling and completely high.

Syd and Cam walked out of resus with the stretcher and Syd inhaled the crisp night air.

'You happy with that then?' he asked as Cam rolled the clunky stretcher into the back of the ambulance.

'Sure thing. Was spot on, son. I only wished that lil' wanker junior doc would wind his neck in.'

'Ah, he's just trying to show off a bit by making us look like dopes. But no such luck on this occasion little ginger man!' said Syd. 'Some people just need to learn that we're all on the same side.'

'Ooh look at you go, Mister Smarty! Too bad they're not testin' you on the grand master plan at your next assessment,' Cam said sarcastically as he sped out of the hospital then immediately returned to his usual driving-Miss-Daisy style over the familiar bumps of the city's roads.

**

On the opposite side of the hospital, Amber's

pass card beeped her through into the staff car park. She pulled on the handbrake and texted Syd to find out where he was.

20:15 hrs – Bravo Unit 989

Soon after vacating the hospital car park, the scratchy voice of a communications operator sounded on the UHF radio, requesting Syd and Cam's truck number. 'Bravo 989?'

Syd, back in the passenger seat, picked up the radio handpiece. 'Bravo 989.'

'Bravo 989. Urgent call. Is your location near Summer Street, Coorparoo?' The operator sounded young and slightly panicked.

The UHF radios used by the service for emergency and daily communications bordered on a joke. Sure they worked, most of the time, but they were a constant bugbear to any of the operational staff attempting to communicate successfully.

Particularly the handheld radios. Fortunately, this was not one of those times: the signal was good and transmissions came through clearly.

Syd wasted no time. 'Bravo 989. We are two streets away from that location. Put us on case and tell us what you know so far.' He spoke quickly and with authority and felt that familiar buzz as his adrenal glands started to release their hormones into his blood.

A different woman took over, perhaps a senior comms operator. Syd could almost taste her voice – bitter as a lemon, rind included, with a side shot of white vinegar.

'Bravo 989, you are going code one to 47 Summer Street, Coorparoo, 27D3, male of unknown age, stab wound to chest, police on scene, Alpha 049 are going code one from the Valley. Please provide timely SITREP once you're on scene.'

'Roger,' Syd said, and whacked the handpiece back in its bracket.

'Can you type it into the GPS, mate?' asked Cam.

'It's the first right then second left, Cam. Let's go.'

Cam paused, looked at the dash in front of Syd, shook his head as if to wake himself up, then flicked on the flashing lights before speeding toward the next street. 'Syd, son, how the hell do you know the location? Have you moved out here or something?'

Syd gathered his stethoscope and squeezed his hands into a pair of nitrile gloves, then chose a pair in Cam's size and rested them on the gearstick for easy access.

'Amber lives not far from here, I know the area pretty well—' Syd leant forward and touched the dash with a sudden realisation, 'Jesus, I could be wrong!' then he reached for the GPS, which was fastened to the dash on a swivel between the two paramedics.

'Don't worry 'bout it mate, we're here. The street looks like a fookin' Christmas tree.'

Cam was right. There were three police cars outside one house and another one further down the road, all stationary with their lights revolving. Syd could see the glow of police flashlights at the front and back of surrounding houses.

The inhabitants of Summer Street were wealthy. Spreading jacaranda trees met above the road, providing cool relief in the hotter months. The houses were large, a few ostentatiously so, and most were a fair distance from the street. The gardens, all illuminated alternately in red and blue, were perfectly manicured.

Cameron drove carefully towards number 47, stopped against a kerb and lowered his window. 'Are we safe to go in?' he said to the nearest police officer.

'We haven't found the assailant yet. The woman inside said he definitely ran down the street.'

Cam turned all the spotlights on, lighting up the

usually quiet street, and scanned the road and footpath ahead, then looked at Syd. 'There's enough coppers here. If you're happy to go in, I am.'

'Yep, let's go,' Syd said, jumping out of the ambulance and opening the storage space behind. He loaded himself up with the airway and oxygen kits, and Cam followed carrying the defibrillator, drug and trauma kits. They crossed the crunchy gravel driveway, passing the hedge, the freshly clipped lawn surrounding the fountain, and feeling the chill of the night as dew covered the toes of their boots. Syd asked another police officer, 'Are you sure it's safe?'

'We've been inside, and the offender has not been located. I'll take you inside though.' She pointed her torch up the harlequin-patterned porch tiles, lighting up a long line of increasingly sized blood drops. 'Watch that' she said. She opened the front door, turned to Syd and said, 'There you go.'

Syd stood on the 'Welcome' doormat, his eyes widening as he took in the room in front of him: the light, the mix of modern and art deco decor, with black and whites of James Cagney and Jean Harlow hanging on the walls. An unmistakable smack of dread hit him then immediately faded.

Syd realised he could see himself, as well as Cam standing behind him. A strange place to put a mirror, he thought, particularly one that took up the entire wall adjacent to the entrance. It did increase the room's size though.

He stepped into the room. A man was on his knees, his eyes wide, face pale and dripping with sweat. He grabbed Syd's leg desperately and gasped, 'Help – me – breathe.'

He leant down to the man, then knelt beside him, preparing the bag valve mask and oxygen kit. Syd registered the shrieking sobs of a woman, glanced up and saw a pretty blonde with bobbed hair, standing beside the police officer.

'What's happened ma'am?' he asked sharply, hoping for an immediate response.

'He said … he … I don't know … he's, he's been stabbed!' she cried, and then burst into fresh tears.

'Cam, cut his shirt off,' Syd instructed, still preparing the oxygen.

Within seconds, the man's chest was exposed and Syd saw one small laceration in the centre of his chest, between his nipples. No visible blood. 'ICPs are on their way?' Syd asked Cam.

'Thank fook,' Cam replied, taking the patient's vital signs.

'I think maybe it's better to keep him sitting up, Cam, yeah?'

'Depends what the knife has hit, and its size,' Cam replied before turning to the woman. 'Ma'am, do you know where the knife is?'

She ignored Cam and continued to sob and wail. The police officer shrugged. 'We haven't found it so far.'

'Could've hit his heart. So we'll just monitor till the ICPs get here. I'll get access now.' Cam threw apart the drug kit and started to prepare for cannulation.

'Sir, stay with me. Sir? Sir!' Syd jammed the ear tips of the stethoscope into his ears and listened to the breathing of his rapidly crashing patient. He felt the patient's weight pressing against him and his head lolled as he slipped into unconsciousness. 'Cam, he's going down. You get set up there for me; I'll stay at the head.'

Syd laid the patient down as the woman began to moan, 'Ken, Ken …'

'Miss, Police, can you or one of your colleagues prepare to guide the other paramedics in the Forester straight in here please,' Syd said, turning back to his patient, whom he now knew as Ken.

Ken's eyes were fluttering, the profuse sweating had ceased, and his face was a new greyer shade of pale. Syd held the bag valve mask firmly against his patient's mouth, flexing his jaw forward for a good fit, and giving gentle breaths of 100 per cent oxygen. Syd noted the rise and fall of Ken's chest, then checked for a carotid pulse. None. He grabbed the opened airway kit and pulled out and fitted a small piece of hard, curved clear plastic into Ken's mouth to depress his tongue and manage his airway then continued to push oxygen into his lungs.

Cam read the ECG and grunted, 'He's in PEA,' then started CPR. 'Fookin' hell man we need to open this guy's chest, decompression, this ain't gonna work, but it's all we can do for now.'

Syd looked at his watch between breaths. It was 20:18. They'd been there for two minutes.

Syd looked at Ken, noted the colour of his skin, on his cheeks, on his neck, on his chest – the wound. What's the chance of someone surviving a stab wound to the chest, he wondered. The statistics? *Out of hospital obviously.* That millisecond of inattention was not only pointless but distracting.

'So, where are we at guys?' Sonia, a short, muscular, attractive intensive care paramedic dropped down beside him, followed by a doctor who introduced herself briefly as Megan.

Syd took a breath to begin his handover but Cam quickly cut in and said, 'Male, unknown age, one stab wound to central chest, about fourth or fifth intercostal space, as you can see.' Cam then tilted his hands away to reveal the wound, which showed a rim of bright red blood with each compression. 'Conscious on arrival, went down less than one minute ago, OPA is in, BVM at 15 litres, no cannulation yet, no other injuries that we have seen.'

'Okay, thanks, just keep on with that while I look around,' said Sonia, as she knelt down and studied Ken's chest and abdomen, paying particular attention around Cam's hands, near the leaking wound. She then felt the patient's neck, front and back, and looked at her gloved hands, seeing no blood, then stood up and spoke in Megan's ear.

Megan said something to Sonia, who then turned back to the patient and listened to Ken's chest through her stethoscope. Megan had whipped out her mobile phone and was chatting, presumably, to the medical manager, who unfortunately was not here. Syd had had the pleasure of seeing this guy in action a few times in the last few months, and was impressed by the direction he gave and his no-bullshit approach.

Syd felt Sonia's breast on his back as she leaned over him and felt calmed by it.

She said to Megan, 'Air entry clear, full fields.'

Megan snapped her phone shut and told Cam to continue CPR; she was going to perform a thoracotomy.

Syd had little idea what this meant and was unsure how the procedure would help, but was assured by Sonia and her marvellously comforting breasts that he should continue bagging.

Ken lay there, splayed before the paramedics, unconscious, and pulseless. Megan knelt down in front of Syd on the right side of Ken, opening yet another kit with tools Syd had never seen. She took a scalpel and sliced across Ken's chest from one side to the other, revealing quite a thick layer of fat, even though the patient was far from heavy, then cut through the thick tissue and muscles protecting his chest with a pair of stubby-ended scissors called trauma shears. As Ken's chest opened up, his lungs popped out, inflating right before Syd's eyes with each breath of oxygen he pushed in. The doctor felt around in the thoracic cavity and scooped out three handfuls of runny and clotted blood and threw them on the rug nearby. There was a lot of blood.

She had made the slice across his chest a little too high and had to snap one rib down to reach the heart, using the trauma shears again. She scooped out more dark clotted blood and exposed the heart, which had one incision in the right ventricle, less than a centimetre wide. Blood pumped out of the small incision with each heartbeat.

She stapled the hole shut with two clumsy staples, but she knew it was too late. It is rare for someone to make it through all of that 'surgery' in an emergency situation.

Ken was dead.

They declared at 20:25 hours.

Everybody else took a breath.

Syd heard Ken's wife crying outside. He looked over at his patient. His heart was still beating. Well, it was beating, but erratically. The rhythm of a dying heart.

Sonia the ICP noticed Syd looking at the heart. 'What are you thinking? she said.

'It's pretty startling to see a beating heart,' said

Sydney, fascinated.

'It's pretty rare to see one, or to even be in this situation, really, in Brisbane anyway,' Sonia said quietly. 'Do you want to touch it?'

Syd was curious, but then he thought his colleagues might think him peculiar for wanting to feel an actual beating heart, albeit a dying and soon to be dead heart. After searching Sonia's clear blue eyes for any judgement, and seeing none, he reached over and put his whole hand around the fitting, dying heart. The soft scent of drifting metallic was everywhere.

Almost at once, a mobile phone began to vibrate on the dining table, buzzing away, demanding attention. The paramedics looked over towards it, then ignored it.

Ken's heart was only pumping due to the cardiac muscles knowing nothing other than to contract and relax, as they had been doing every second of every day for the last forty-nine years.

Syd sat beside Ken solemnly gazing at the heart. It had felt like nothing he had felt before. He had been around the innards of animals killed for food when he was living and working on farms in his earlier years, but this was utterly different. The human heart in his hand was a smooth muscle the size of his fist, but when it tried to work it was more taut than the strongest muscle he had ever felt.

A human heart, in the palm of his hand: not fully

functioning, but thrilling. Remarkable.

He took another deep breath and held it. His neck thumped by his own beating heart. One drop of sweat fell from the tip of his nose and mixed with a small puddle of blood in the dead man's chest cavity.

That was enough.

Two weeks earlier – Ken

The hallway was filled with suits. Some cheap, some luxurious, but all of them covering a human with questionable morals. They strutted about, shaking hands and smiling confidently, although they would only be buddies when no cameras were there to film them.

This was State Parliament.

Probably not *all* of the members had dubious morals, but some most certainly did, and they disguised it effortlessly as though they'd been doing it forever.

It was their first morning break, and the best local coffee business had been hired to provide finely made pastries and coffees for the morning's sitting.

In addition to being state elected officials who demanded grandeur and insisted on the appearance of nobility, they were also coffee connoisseurs.

The Honourable Neville Nelson – broad chested, pompous and red faced – flashed his dirty teeth in a fake smile. Most people knew there was trouble ahead if he grasped your arm when he shook your hand. The last person he'd done that to was his assistant, a young woman named Kelly. Reportedly, he was having an affair with Kelly and she wanted out.

One Friday afternoon, in front of all the staff, he shook her hand with the empty sincerity of the arm grab. On the following Monday he had the paperwork to prove Kelly had been misappropriating funds. She was found guilty almost immediately of misusing her fuel card. She'd never work in the public sector again.

Kelly had been replaced with Ken. And although the Honourable Neville Nelson didn't have an affair with Ken in mind when he hired him, he most certainly had other indecorous ideas.

The Honourable Neville Nelson had Ken worked out from the start of the interview as a hard-working, crowd-pleasing, subservient man who would do anything to win the approval of his domineering boss.

The Honourable Neville Nelson knew how to read people.

On Ken's first Thursday, the Honourable Neville Nelson invited Ken and his wife to his Gold Coast apartment for a 'get to know you' weekend. Unfortunately for Ken, his wife couldn't attend and Ken spent the weekend in a haze of hallucinogenic debauchery.

He would never speak of this to his wife. He would not tell the few friends he had, and most definitely he would tell no one at work. It was the deepest secret of his life, one that could never be revealed. But he continued to follow the Honourable Neville Nelson around, doing what he did best, being agreeable.

After rushing down a half-cup of caramel latte, Ken advised the Honourable Neville Nelson he would be going to the bathroom. Such detail was probably not warranted, but the Honourable Neville Nelson usually appreciated it, and said he needed to go as well.

The two gentlemen entered the expanse of the dark-tiled bathroom, and the chitter-chatter and teaspoon clinking ceased completely as the heavy door swung shut.

Ken approached the urinal, his leather-soled business shoes pattering, and lowered his fly. The Honourable Neville Nelson pushed on the stall doors to check they were empty. They were.

The Honourable Neville Nelson stood behind Ken, about a metre away.

'So, I've been talking with Peter and Paul – ahh jeez, that sounds like the bloody disciples doesn't it?' Nelson snorted. 'Anyway, we'll have to be quick. I need you to do a pickup tonight, like last time, but for six of us this time. Can you organise that?'

Ken hadn't even started to urinate, but had been standing there for long enough he felt he should have been finished by now, and pretended so.

'Ah, well, if that's what you'd like, I'm going to have to chat with our contact,' he said, pretending to shake, 'I don't know how much that will be—'

'Don't worry about the money, mate, we'll fix you up after. What it costs, it costs. And we trust you anyway. I don't even *have* contact with *our contact*, it's just too risky – you know that. And the lads are bringing their wives this time. Plus, someone special.' The Honourable Neville Nelson's inflection didn't sound honourable at all.

'Are you having another party this weekend?'

'Sure am, mate. And you're invited!'

Ken turned around. 'Thank you Mr Nelson, but I cannot attend this time. My wife and I have plans.'

'You can bring her too if you like.'

'Thank you, again, but I just don't think she's into that sort of thing.'

20:25 hrs – Lorraine

Lorraine sat at a small table in the middle of her kitchen. Although modest, her house was furnished graciously, with a style that reflected her own tranquil nature. She stared at the wall, wondering more about herself than Bradley, whose life she had decided to end.

She wondered why she had been given this addiction. To being thrilled. To being excited, to the surge of adrenaline. The controlled anxiety. The focus. The flutter of the heart. The prickle of sweat.

When she switched Bradley's drugs, she knew she had, essentially, killed a man. It was only a matter of time. She felt calm, for now.

On the table sat a bulky, thick book: *Organic*

Chemistry of Drug Degradation. She knew the topic well and had recently learnt even more. She read over three key paragraphs without touching the table or the book. She grinned. 'And that's what you'll get, shithead.'

Lorraine reached for her mobile phone and tapped her mother's contact photo. She needed to tell her the recent development in her plan. She had to vent, and her mother was the only person she would tell the details to. They had crossed many metaphorical boundaries and borders together – walking away from Heather's second abusive husband; helping Lorraine learn to manage her addictive personality – and were far more enmeshed than most mothers and daughters. They had similar personalities, and similar hobbies.

This time, though, the phone rang out and went to voice mail. Lorraine turned her phone off and continued to sit and stare.

Lorraine's mother stood outside her own house, crying.

20:35 hrs – 43 Ferguson Skyline Drive, Seven Hills

'That was just delicious. Thank you, my love,' Ted said as he quietly laid his knife and fork across his empty plate. He touched his wife's arm, causing her to drop the forkful of carefully balanced peas.

'Well, it was a team effort, love. Now let me get through mine,' she said.

'Sorry about that, love. Great dinner though. Chops 'n' vegies, what a classic. Does us good.'

Audrey mumbled agreement as she set about capturing the evasive peas once more.

The couple sat at the dining table that only just fitted the room. They loved the table. It was a family heirloom and, despite its impracticality in such a small space, they had learned to work with it. A television sat on a nearby kitchen bench and a ceiling-high cabinet of glassware had been moved to the adjoining living room beside the couch. Framed family photos sat on the lower shelves.

'I'll wash these up,' said Ted once Audrey had finished.

'Okay. Thank you, love. Actually, no, just use the dishwasher, it's almost full now,' Audrey said.

'I think it's better for my back if I wash up, dear. Bending down to fill up that machine gives me grief to no end.'

'Oh. Well, I'll do it then, love.'

'No, love, we can both do it. I could pass the dishes down to you after I give them a rinse.'

'That sounds just grand. Another team effort,' she said.

After the dishwasher was packed and switched on, Ted waddled over and read yesterday's newspaper for five minutes. Audrey switched on the television, flicked through the channels and, as usual, was disappointed with the programs she found. She switched it off.

Each of them did what they wanted, but they were always together. They didn't always speak to each other, but when they did, it was with respect and politeness.

They both completed the necessary bathroom

duties, before retiring to the bedroom and changing into their nightwear.

'How are you feeling, love?' Ted asked.

'Feeling good, no problems,' said Audrey.

Ted walked around to Audrey's side of the bed and gave her a courteous kiss. 'Thanks for tonight Auds.'

Audrey chuckled. 'Oh, *what for* you big slobbery dog?' she said sweetly.

'Just for being you. And for loving me.'

'You too, love,' Audrey replied, 'and don't forget – sixty years next Tuesday. We're going to have everybody here for the weekend too.'

'I know, I know,' said Ted as he walked back around the bed, 'I can't believe it's been sixty years already.'

The two of them inched into bed and lay on their backs.

'It's going to be a good weekend,' said Ted, looking at the ceiling before switching off the light. 'Good night, my love.'

'Good night, precious heart.'

Twenty years earlier – Sydney

Sydney sat on the back doorstep in the shade attempting to eat, rather than drink, a rapidly melting ice block. He had a face full of freckles and a head of shaggy hair, and he passionately disliked having it cut. He still wore his private boys' school uniform on this Friday afternoon, but had removed his shoes. Hair was a constant source of dispute between himself, the school, and his mother, who always followed the school rules. Sydney, predictably, lost the argument every time and detested having to conform, even at such a young age.

Michael, Sydney's father, walked out of the

house and sat next to his young son. 'Blimey, it's hot in there. Much nicer out here,' he said. 'So, what should we get up to this weekend?'

Sydney knew he could ask for pretty much whatever he wanted, and, within reason, he'd get it. He spent every second weekend with his father, who spoiled him rotten. Michael felt this made up for the mistakes he had made with Sydney's mother.

'I wanna kick the footy.' He looked up to his dad. 'Oh, and the Masters of the Universe show at the exhibition centre is on tomorrow and Sunday … that would be great! Can we go? Can we?'

Michael smiled and said, 'Well, we can kick the footy later when it cools down a bit, but only if you pronounce your words correctly.'

Syd drank the remaining gaudy green slush. 'I don't remember what I said.'

'I wanna.'

'Oh, then I meant I *want* to, actually, no, I would *like* to, very much please,' Syd said cheekily.

'Well in that case, dear sir, we may be able to do so, but only because you spoke so finely.' Michael said in an aristocratic English accent. 'And I think, by the power of Grayskull, we could probably go and visit He-Man tomorrow morning, after you're well rested from a big sleep tonight.'

Sydney wriggled with excitement then proceeded to rattle off the names and personalities of each of the Masters of the Universe figurines he owned. He dropped the hint at least five times that he didn't yet own Skeletor and couldn't wait to slot the Leader of the Evil Warriors into his scenario.

'We'll see what we can do,' Michael said. They grinned at each other.

'I'm gonna get the footy and practise my passes,' said Syd as he raced inside.

'I beg your pardon?'

'I mean, I'm *going* to get the footy and practise,' Syd said from his room.

Two minutes passed before Syd returned to the back step, his eyes wide. Before he could speak, Michael said kindly, 'Where's the footy, you goose?'

'Dad, there's some police at the front door. I said I'd come and get you.'

Michael sighed deeply, got to his feet and walked past Sydney. 'Stay here please,' he said.

Syd did as he was told, for about five seconds, then he raced outside and around the back corner of the house, spying out to the police car, which was parked on the other side of the street.

Stacey, Michael's current wife of around five years, sat in the back of the police car. Syd could see she was clearly upset and crying into her hands. He toyed with the idea of sneaking over and checking on her, but thought better of it. He didn't want to be known as 'the eight-year-old who tried to outsmart the police'.

Soon Michael returned to the back step. Syd

perched on the railing, waiting for a report. 'What's happened Dad?' he said.

Michael looked meek and defeated. 'Well, I have to go with your stepmother and speak with the police.' His shoulders dropped. 'I have to call your mum to come and get you. I'm sorry buddy.'

'Why is Stacey crying?' Syd asked.

Michael left what seemed an endless pause. 'Because she doesn't love me anymore.'

Fifteen minutes later, Syd's mum arrived, completely ignored Michael as well as the police, took Syd's hand and led him gently to her car before driving off slowly.

Syd didn't understand what happened that day, but the memory of it had buried deep.

Over the next few months, on the rare and inconsistent occasions when he did see his father, Syd pestered him to explain what had happened that day. His father only ever replied with vague comments such as, 'She fell out of love with me', and despite Syd's constant questioning, he was never answered with a better reply.

Over the next few years, Syd began to bother his mother for the details of what had led to their divorce when Syd was just 3 years old. In due course, she told him the full story. Which, of course, was an understated account of domestic violence.

21:15 hrs – 47 Summer Street, Coorparoo

For the next forty-five minutes, the three paramedics sat at the living-room table, quietly discussing the events that had just taken place. Ken's body lay nearby, opened across the chest like a carcass, its shape clearly defined under the hospital linen the paramedics had draped over it.

Sonia asked Syd if he felt okay doing the paperwork there while a corpse changed colour under the starched sheet.

'I'm okay,' he said. 'Thanks. It'll be fine.' He appreciated the care shown by his senior colleagues.

Syd and Cam crossed the t's and dotted the i's on the paperwork while Sonia packed up what little gear she had used. Megan soon returned, strolling casually past the body and signalling to Sonia with a hammy wink and head tilt to follow her.

'I've been speaking with the police and the wife. Looks like a 'wrong place, wrong time' type incident. The wife doesn't know anything. The cops say the patient's untouched wallet is in the car, which is unlocked, and the car key was still in his tracksuit pocket. So it's all a bit of a mystery really.' Megan pressed both fists down on the table, apparently more interested in taking on the role of detective than pondering the fact that she had just cut a man open like Braveheart. She continued piecing the puzzle together. 'Maybe it's political. He *is* an assistant to a member of parliament.'

She noticed Syd. 'Are you okay Sydney?' she asked.

'Yeah I'm okay,' Syd spoke firmly, 'but I'm just wondering what else we, or you, could have done for him.'

The doctor pushed up from the table and stood straight. 'There are so many variables with stab wounds to the chest, and it's very difficult to say what could be done. In this gentleman's case, aside from what we did, there isn't much else that could've been done for him. A finger into the wound blocking the hole in the heart might work sometimes, but usually only in the movies. Out of hospital, and with the angle of penetration of this patient's stab wound, there's really nothing else that could be done. What we attempted here is often successful in theatre, but not so much in the field.'

Syd gave her a searching look. Megan continued. 'So, the answer to your question, Sydney, is *not much else*. You did what you could, what you were supposed to do, and you did it in a very calm and controlled manner. Even though it's not such a good evening for our patient, you did well.'

Syd stirred in his seat, uncomfortable with the praise.

'Have you got family and friends to speak with if this affects you in a way that you don't expect?' she asked.

'Thanks, I think I'll be okay. I can talk with my girlfriend; she's been a nurse for a few years and has seen a fair bit. And Cam of course.'

He looked to Cam, who nodded and replied with a booming 'Aye'.

'And if it stresses me out I'll give the work counsellors a call. No problems.'

Syd was glad he had managed to deliver his statements with confidence, despite Ken's wailing wife who could be heard through the door crying and sobbing.

Soon the paramedics had finished their paperwork and had signatures from the senior members, which was always made out to be a big deal in cases like this one. Megan led the way outside, followed in order of seniority by Sonia, Cameron, and Sydney. They walked slowly, respectfully, through the yellow police cordon tape, each of the paramedics giving the wife a sincere sombre look as they passed: Sonia sad, Cameron cast down, Syd stressed. The wife touched his arm then suddenly forced him into a tight hug. The iPad fell from his hands and the screen cracked as it bounced on the footpath. The fresh clean scent of expensive shampoo drifted about as the blonde bob pushed against his chest.

Sonia and Cameron spun around. Syd looked at them both, wide-eyed, then instinctively wrapped both his arms around her and said, 'I wish I had the words.' His eyes began to sting as she sobbed into his shirt and he squeezed them shut as he leant his head down to her luxuriously soft hair. Whether or not Ken's wife knew why Ken had been stabbed made no difference to Syd. He pulled her in close. *Life is too short.*

He looked at Sonia, who stood staring with dropped jaw. Cameron started to move back towards Syd; he knew the potential effect of trauma being unintentionally passed on by a patient's family. He reached out and held the wife's elbow, which was wrapped tightly round Syd's flank.

'Ma'am, my deepest condolences,' he said with Scottish sincerity, 'but we have to go now.'

They probably didn't have to go, but Cam used it

as a classic excuse to pry them out of sticky situations.

'My name is Heather. I just want to give him one last hug,' she said. Syd let go of her, but she had not fully released him from her grip.

'You mean Ken, right? Not me.'

As soon as the tactless sentence left his lips, Syd shuddered. She took a small step back from him, still keeping him close, and looked up into his wet eyes, then let out a loud hysterical cackling laugh. Sonia quickly stepped in front of Cameron, grabbed Syd by the elbow and signalled for him to follow her immediately. They walked back to the vehicles, leaving Cam with Ken's crying wife, a couple of coppers, and a broken iPad.

Fifteen years earlier – Heather and Lorraine

Heather tapped down her front path as Lorraine skipped along behind. They had spent the night at the house of Heather's best friend and her daughter, after the four of them had attended a musical in the city.

The chill bit at them, and clouds made the day look closer to dusk than noon. Mild smog and the dampness of an approaching storm filled their nostrils.

'Hakuna matata … what a wonderful phrase … hakuna matata …. da da daa da da da,' Lorraine sang over the distant rumble of thunder. A train clanked along behind the townhouse where they lived in North Sydney, leaving not a sense idle.

Heather pushed in the key and Lorraine ran up and hugged her leg.

'That show last night was so fantastic, Mum, I want to go again. Can we go again please?'

'It was good wasn't it?' Heather said. 'But you may have to save up some pocket money before we can go again, honey.'

Lorraine let go and looked up at her mother. 'And Dad can come next time, too. Oh I can't wait to tell Dad about it. I think he'll love it!'

Heather pushed open the door and Lorraine sprinted inside towards the kitchen. 'Dad, Dad! Where are you Dad?' Lorraine's sneakers squeaked on the parquet as she sped around searching for her father. 'Daaa-a-d? Hello?'

Heather strolled to the kitchen and turned on the kettle while Lorraine bounded up the stairs without losing a beat as she continued to sing. Heather stood and leant both hands on the counter and closed her eyes. She felt a strange sense of dread, and leant on the bench, feeling suddenly dizzy. She was gathering herself when a horrible thought occurred to her.

At the same moment the thought entered her mind, she heard an ear-splitting scream from Lorraine upstairs. Instantly she turned and ran, leaping four stairs at a time, into the main bedroom where her daughter stood, shocked and sobbing. In front of Lorraine, her father sat on the carpet, leaning against the bedside table in his usual jeans and shirt. His eyes were closed, his mouth was slightly open and dry, his head rested against the bed. In his left forearm, a hypodermic syringe was embedded in a vein, with the plunger fully depressed.

His skin was pale and cold. Both Heather and Lorraine recoiled when they first knelt down and held him through their sobs and tears. It didn't feel like the man they had known and loved.

His big laugh and the giggles he had provoked with his 'dad jokes' seemed to echo in the room as they clung to the memories of the man they had loved: his proposal to Heather eleven years earlier while they sailed amongst a thousand Indonesian islands; teaching Lorraine science and maths well beyond the ability of her peers; their shared love of learning; the memory techniques he had taught her, so that she had memorised the periodic table, completely, by the age of seven. The three of them, together, had run on the beaches of Manly, knowing all the lifeguards after Lorraine and her team had won the Nippers championships for the last two years.

They knew everybody. They were the happy family. They were the family who were good at everything. They were the family that everybody envied.

Heather and Lorraine held each other for an hour before Heather called the police.

21:30 hrs – Bravo 989

'You mean Ken right, not me?' Syd sat in the passenger seat and buried his face in his hands. 'What the hell was I thinking?'

'Ah, don't worry about it too much, son. It's all learning, ain't it?'

'I suppose you could say learning. Or just complete humiliation!'

'I'm serious. Remember it; yes. But don't be too hard on yourself for it, right?'

'Cam, that was a pretty sad job. I really feel sorry for the wife.'

'Yes, lad, I agree,' said Cam, 'but maybe it was a good thing she was there for his final moments. Maybe not. Either way, it's a shitty situation that is way outside our control. We helped as much as we could.' Cam continued to drive through the mild evening traffic and realised he may have sounded heartless. 'Have you ever lost someone close to you, son?' he asked kindly.

Syd paused. 'A mate. About six or seven years ago now. We jackarooed together on a sheep station in New South for two years. I suppose we were kind of close. After I'd left that job and moved to my family farm, he'd been promoted to head stockman.' Syd spoke slowly, pausing now and then. 'Horse-riding accident. No one saw it. And he was a good rider, too. After mustering all day, he and I used to race our horses back from the yards to the homestead. Whoever lost unsaddled the nags; whoever won got the beers ready,' Syd recalled. 'Bloody sad funeral.'

'Young funerals … eh.'

'Eh?'

'They're the worst. Unexpected. No one expects a kid to die.'

'True. But I bet you that guy just then, Ken, didn't wake up this morning expecting to die today.'

'You're right. But that's work, isn't it. We *should* care, but we *have* to care to the *exact right degree*,' said Cam. 'When everything's new and exciting and memorable, it's great, but I don't want you to go crazy while it's all being processed in your heart and mind, right?'

'I won't go crazy, Cam. I'm already there!'

'Sorry mate, I shouldn't have asked if you'd lost someone; none of my business.'

'Actually, Cam, it *is* your business. You're my mentor and I'm your student, so we *have* to know each other's business to look after each other and be a good team.'

'I know.' Cam was smiling. 'I know you're a crazy Aussie who speaks another language sometimes—'

'That's rich coming from a Scot!' Syd said.

'And we're a' Jock Tamson's bairns!' Cam laid the accent on as thick as possible.

'Yeah, now you're doing it on purpose!'

'Aye. I can't always speak Australian ye know?'

'So, what's it mean?'

'What's what mean?'

'The Jack Thompson thing?'

'Ah, ha ha, it's *we're a' Jock Tamson's bairns*. Means we're all the same in the end.'

'Could've just said that,' said Syd, grinning.

'So what's the jackarooin' about?' asked Cam.

'Working on a sheep or cattle station, riding horses pretty much every day, mustering then working the stock, fixing fences, motorbikes ... jack of all trades really, but the learner version. *Country stuff*, Cam.'

'I know you're a country boy.' He looked over at Syd. 'And a damn shame about your mate.'

'Definitely sad. Man we had some fun though. We were pretty much at the same level on most things, you know? So we were kind of in competition with each other all the time. It was good. Like having a brother. Trying to outdo each other. We'd both had a year horse riding and were quite good at reading stock movements, and whip cracking, and shearing sheep when we had to. Oh god, now that is the most difficult work I have ever done, no doubt about it.' Syd looked out at the city shops whirring past. 'He was a better shot than I was, but I reckon I always outdid him on the horses.'

'You got some good memories, mate.'

'For sure.'

Darkness had enveloped the city and low trailing clouds were veiling the moon. The ambulance followed the speed limit exactly.

'So how's the woman?' said Cam.

'She seemed pretty bloody upset to me. Didn't you notice?'

Cam looked over at Syd to see if he had actually misunderstood his question. He had. 'I mean *your* woman, you donkey.'

'Oh! *My* woman. Like *I own her*, yes,' Syd replied mockingly. 'Yep, she's great. No, actually she's okay. Actually, she was acting a bit strange earlier tonight on the phone. Not sure about that. But all in all, she's great. I love her, man. Why's that?'

'Just askin' mate. They're all a bit strange you know. In a good way. Mostly.'

'Hmm, way to commit to a statement Cam,' Syd said sarcastically. 'What's strange about Claire?'

'Ah nah, she's all right. She's a fine, fiery, traditional Scottish lass with good morals and an even better eye for a fine gentleman.'

'So what's she doing with you?' Syd asked predictably.

Cam ignored him. 'But the women these days, son, I don't know how you keep up with them. I watched this TV series called—'

'Not everybody is like the movies, Cam. And why are you talking like you're ninety-five? Aren't you only ten years older than me?'

'Somethin' like that. Aye … I'm thirty-eight you wee lad.'

'Well stop talking like an old grump.'

'So you don't think there's anything strange about how quickly everybody wants to show as much of themselves as they can these days? I just don't get it.'

'You mean the way people dress? Or how everybody *bares their soul* on the internet? What are you talking about, Ol' Scotsman?'

'Yeah, I suppose I sound like an old fart don't I?' Cam said, relinquishing his point. He drove on for a short time before breaking the silence. 'It's just as though everybody has got this out-bloody-rageous loud voice and everybody else has to hear it. That's what I'm saying.'

'Loud voice? As in, social media?'

'Yep.'

'*You're* on Facebook. What are you talking about?'

'That's how I know, son. And Claire made me get it anyway. But there is so much rubbish on it. Sometimes I wonder why they need it all.'

'Cam, I don't get it either. Although I must admit I *do* like Facebook. It's as though I can know what people are doing, and care or 'like' it from a distance, but I don't have to care too much.'

Cam left a purposeful silence, hoping Syd would click to it. They both opened their mouths to speak at the same time, and Cam hesitated.

'And that's how I should be with work, right?' said Syd.

'When it comes to your heart, at work, yes, son. It's self-preservation.'

Back at the station, the two paramedics restocked the ambulance and the kits. They were not yet inside the 'meal-break time window', but Syd, for once, actually wanted to be left alone for some time and not called out. He felt tired; his mind needed a break.

They sat on an armchair each and clacked the recliner legs up at the same time.

As Cam turned on the television, Syd put his earphones in and fell asleep almost immediately listening to an acoustic guitar playing a song on the sea. He dreamed a strange but comforting dream, one that lingered after he woke, as if it had carried some special meaning.

Syd woke sharply, and smiled. He felt the vibration on his hip and realised the smile was wasted on this wake-up call.

'Aaah!' Cam boomed as he read his pager. 'This'll be a right load of shite then. It's out at Greenslopes. You want me on this one, son?'
Syd shook his head to clear it. 'Nah, thanks Cam, I'll do it. Have to get that systematic approach perfected, remember.'

21:55 hrs – 509 Upper Cedar Street, Greenslopes

'Hello, ambulance,' Syd said through the closed security door. He heard movement somewhere inside. 'Just a sec, I think the paramedics are here.' The voice was female. A thin, well-dressed, black-haired woman appeared at the door with a mobile phone in one hand and a glass of red wine in the other.

She smiled. 'Ah hello, that didn't take long. You guys are so quick. It's open.' The two paramedics entered. 'It's my daughter, the youngest one. I don't know what to do. She's in her bedroom crying and she's been there all afternoon and evening. One of her friends somehow got my number and texted me.

Apparently she'd told him she was going to do something tonight that would *end the pain*.'

'Okay then,' said Syd, taking in the family photos on the walls and trophies lining the bookcase. 'Well, my name's Sydney and this is Cameron.' Cam waved and smiled. 'What's your daughter's name?'

'Hold on, darling, I have to speak with these paramedics, can I call you back?' she asked the phone. Syd raised both eyebrows. 'Okay darling, I'm very much looking forward to it. Chat soon, bye.' She turned her attention to Syd. 'I'm sorry Simon, what did you say?'

Syd faked a smile. 'I asked what your daughter's name is? And my name is Sydney.'

'Oh please do excuse me Sydney. Her name is Riley.' This time Syd detected a slight slur.

'How old is Riley?'

'Fourteen in July.'

'What is Riley's medical history?'

'She suffers panic attacks and has had depression for the last year. She sees Doctor Rafter at the PA.'

'I don't know Doctor Rafter. Is Riley on any medications?'

'She's taking Prozac.'

'Has she been on Prozac for the whole year? Has she made any threats to you about anything else tonight?'

'Last year, she started off by taking my antidepressants because she said she was down. I thought that was dangerous so I took her to the shrink who got her on her own script. And no, I haven't seen her for the last half hour. She's in her room. She said she didn't want dinner, so we ate without her.'

The mother then led Syd and Cam past the dinner table, with four places set. Three had half eaten servings of rib-eye steaks topped with pesto and a side of grilled asparagus. It looked cold. There were two glass bowls of delicate salads in the middle of the table. It appeared that the three people who had begun eating had disappeared halfway through the meal.

'Continue on guys, this shouldn't take too long,' said the mother as she passed the table.

'I beg your pardon ma'am?' said Syd as he followed her. 'Were you talking to me?'

'No no no, just organising things in my head for tomorrow, that's all,' she replied in a chirpy tone.

They walked to the back of the house past four closed doors until the mother knocked on a door with a neatly decorated 'R'.

'Riley? Riley?' the mother said softly. 'The paramedics are here to see you honey. Can I open the door?' There was no answer. 'We took the locks off a few months ago. You know, just in case,' the mother whispered to Syd. 'Okay Riley, we're coming in.'

She turned the door handle slowly and pressed

her hand and face against the door, as if attempting to dramatise the act even further; she'd clearly seen way too many horror films. As the door opened, as if in slow motion, Syd saw a young, pretty, pale-faced girl sitting on her zebra print bedspread looking up at the three adults before her. She was breathing abnormally quickly.

'I know you don't want to talk, honey, but I thought these guys could chat with you, and help with what has happened to your fingers, because you said they were sore didn't you darling? Or tingling? Riley?' The girl ignored her mother and immediately turned her back. The room was pink, black and white, and looked as perfect as the photos in a renovation magazine – not a thing out of place. On one black wall, letters spelt out 'RILEY' in the same style as the R on the door. White bookshelves flanked the double bed and there was a big black and white photo of Riley with her mother and another girl smiling at the beach. Nearby was a similar photo of Riley on her own. On the shelves were small, colour-coordinated boxes, each perfectly placed, and the dimmed lighting of the bedside lamp added to the orderly and impressive effect.

'Hi Riley. I'm Sydney, and this is Cameron. Your mum's a bit worried about you and we're going to do our best to help, but we'll talk about that in a tick. For now, I need you to control your breathing, yes? Rumour has it you've got tingling in your fingers? Have you still got that?' Syd stepped closer to Riley, held her hand and took her pulse.

The mother made a point of leaving the room, making sure everybody watched her go.

'Rumour has it?' Riley puffed.

'Sorry Riley, I was trying to be funny. So, the reason your fingers and hands are tingling is because of your breathing. You need to slow it down. Only you can fix this, but, I'll give you a hand and talk you through it, okay?'

Riley looked interested and turned to face Syd. 'So, you just have to breathe in threes, okay? In for three,' Syd took a deep breath in, 'hold it for three,' he said while holding it in, 'then out for three,' he said as he released, 'then start all over again. I'm going to stay with you until you get this breathing under control, yeah?' Syd then repeated the breathing exercises as Riley breathed.

Cam had no need to help Syd with the assessment. They both knew this was a problem that overanxious or panicked people commonly experienced, and one that often frustrated paramedics as it could be simply resolved without any medical intervention.

Within four minutes, Riley's hands and fingers felt normal again. 'Oh my god, I can't believe it's, like, better just from changing my breathing,' she said. 'That's pretty cool.'

'Yep it's crazy town, isn't it?' said Syd, trying to

sound young.

Riley sat with her legs crossed and shoulders hunched, playing with her duvet cover, her head down, so Syd switched to Dad mode. 'The body is a perfect container, and it's just what we put into our container that changes it for better or worse.' Cam pretended to cover a giggle.

'Is there anything else we can help you with Riley?'

Syd knew better than to ask this question of people who he had judged to be desperate. The proverb *give them an inch and they'll take a mile* pretty much summed up the hazard of asking open-ended questions and offering help before you understood the issues. Much of the emergency medical profession shared his views, and for good reason. Although Syd had been a paramedic for a short time, he had quickly discovered that there were plenty of people who fell into the *inch-mile* category. He knew it was frowned upon to judge people, to talk about 'categories' of people, but had also identified that people in front-line jobs sometimes needed to think that way. He had to judge. He had to categorise. He had to work out if a patient was emergently sick, or simply needed assistance, or was a threat to himself or his partner; then present an immediate judgement, and act accordingly. He thought of this more as a likable challenge than something to be ashamed of. He knew the platitudes about not judging people didn't fit with the human survival instincts that had evolved over thousands of years, which was why he, and most of his colleagues, would continue to use judgement calls that had proven useful.

Syd was amused by how many people were quick to say 'You can't judge me!' and yet were interested in – almost obsessed by – 'reality' television shows based on people being judged by a panel of 'experts', and usually humiliated before a massive audience.

Syd judged Riley to be one of those inch–mile people, but he knew she was young and had a history of depression, and that she also had what seemed to be a drama-queen of a mother. Her home life too, seemed quite strange. Perhaps a chat would tell him what was actually going on, and then he might be able to help. Predictably, Riley jumped at the chance.

'Well, my last school report sucked, and … like, my parents put a lot of pressure on me to do well – actually it's just my dad, he's, like, the genius of the family, even though he's never here, yeah. He expects big things from me.'

'Where's your dad tonight?'

'Amsterdam, I think. Maybe staying in Dubai, or maybe Singapore. Not sure. Why?'

'Just wondering. Tell me why you were panicking earlier today.'

'My mum was, like, stressing about the most random things at me.' Riley fiddled with a loose thread from her bedding. 'And family dinners are so important apparently, 'cause, like, we have to sit around every night and, like, say what amazing things we achieved today.'

'When you speak with your counsellor, Riley, do you speak with them about how you feel about these kinds of things?'

'I dunno … my mum made me start talking with Marc – he's the counsellor – because of what happened with my sister … she died … that's her up there,' she pointed to the black and white print. 'Always looking down on me aren't you sis? Yeah I suppose she is … anyway, I dunno … I'm just sick of Dad's pressure … Maybe I need to, like, kill myself. That'll shut him up!' She looked down at the loose thread, slowly unpicking it.

Syd saw Cam roll his eyes. 'That's probably not the outcome anybody wants Riley.' Syd knew full well she would have to be transported to hospital now for a mental health assessment. 'Would you like to chat to anybody else about this? It's a big thing to say you're going to kill yourself. Particularly to shut your dad up.'

'Nah. Marc is, like, good to talk to. I don't wanna talk to anyone else.'

'Do you think he's helping you though? Maybe a new set of ears might be what you need?'

Riley was unmoved. 'Maybe …' She looked up into Syd's green eyes, 'but it has to be a man. I, like, can't talk to women.' Her small hands began to tremble.

'No problems,' said Syd, 'but I think that may be a problem in itself. What do you think, Riley?'

The girl took a deep breath, moved towards Syd and swung her feet to the ground.

'You wanna know what I think?' She squinted at Syd and Cam. 'I think my mother has sent you two in here 'cause she has, like, no idea what to do with me. And I think she, like, worries herself stupid since I took a heap of her Zoloft. But I don't wanna, like, let down my dad anymore 'cause, like, he gives me everything and I do wanna be a good daughter. And I think I've gotta not be so … like, like …'

'Indecisive?' asked Syd, unable to help himself.

'Fat!'

'Oh Jesus spare the world, you are not fat.'

'Yeah, that's what my friends say but when I look in the mirror all I see is a huge fat pig!'

Syd took a deep breath. 'Two more questions before I go and get your mum and we head off, Riley. Just relax, there is nothing to be stressed about right now. So, firstly, how have you been sleeping lately?'

'I, like, sleep as much as I can. As soon as I get home I go to sleep. It's been like that, like, for a year or maybe longer.'

'And have you taken any medications that aren't prescribed to you, or any drugs or alcohol in the last twenty-four hours?' Syd asked.

'Nope. Just my Fluoxetine. I haven't touched Mum's stuff. No other drugs. I don't wanna be like that druggo girl, the one that smashes it just to get guys. And alcohol, like, I'm allowed to drink what I want, like, my friends think it's weird, and I don't even really, like ... like it, so I don't drink much. My parents think if they let me, like, have it when I want, that I won't do it behind their backs.'

'Thank you, Riley. I'll go and get your mum, and hopefully we can find you someone to chat with.'
Syd thought it unnecessary to push her about drug use, and particularly the alcohol these parents were happily letting their child consume. He would not bring it up with the mother, just the counsellor. Syd had no idea what the repercussions would be for parents who allowed a thirteen-year-old child to drink alcohol, albeit in the privacy of their own home, but, like Riley's friends, he thought it, 'like', weird.

22:15 hrs - Bradley

Bradley awoke in his car as if from a bad dream. He was sweating profusely and his breathing was shallow and rapid. He felt stabbing pains in his chest and stomach. He raced home, unsure what to do next.

The front door crashed open as he surged through, keys jangling to the percussion of his hyperventilation. Sweat beaded his forehead. He paced past the purple octopus print in the hallway and into the kitchen.

He half-filled a dirty glass with bourbon and slammed most of it down in one gulp. He felt it instantly calm his nerves, as it had frequently throughout his life.

He gazed through the kitchen window at the neighbouring fence and considered his options.

Possibility one: Ken was merely injured and down $7000, stolen by *his drug dealer*. Surely he wouldn't report that? Ken had been the Assistant to the Minister for Health for such a short time, surely his job and reputation would be the most important things to him?

Possibility two: Ken was merely injured and down $7000, stolen by *someone*. He reports it saying he's never seen the assailant before but gives an accurate - if general - description of his drug dealer, who the police may or may not know.

Possibility three: Ken is injured badly, maybe dead, and down $7000, which his wife may or may not know about. She may or may not have known about the deal. She may or may not have told someone else. Or maybe someone else could have seen the whole thing. Maybe.

Bradley realised each possibility led to endless further possibilities, particularly when he didn't know how seriously injured Ken was.

The lack of information unnerved him.

He threw down another half glass of liquor. His hands shook as he plugged a cigarette between his lips and attempted to light it. After four failed attempts with the flint scratching and sparking, Bradley worked out that the lighter was empty and threw it against the kitchen wall with a frustrated

'Fuck!'

Still shaken over having just stabbed a man, Bradley agitatedly marched around his house, trying to calm down while wondering where he could get a simple thing like fire. He longed for a nicotine hit to accompany the bourbon, but also knew there were no more lighters in the house.

Bradley noticed the boxy portable butane gas stove, which looked out of place in his otherwise neat white kitchen. 'That'll work,' he said aloud. He had been using it for the last two days after smelling gas leaking from the stove. He had switched the gas off at the main and called the local gas technicians who were booked for tomorrow.

Bradley turned the knob, heard the click and saw the spitting butane flame. He lit the cigarette, concentrating on steadying his hands. Bradley drew in hard, then exhaled, shoving the kitchen window open to air the room.

The cigarette wasn't enough. He wanted more. He wanted a different feeling. The alcohol had done as much as it could to his brain. Now he wanted to escape reality altogether. Without a second thought, he walked to his bedroom safe, opened it and grabbed the small black plastic case, slamming the safe shut, unaware of anything unusual. Even if there were signs of Lorraine's intrusion, Bradley would not have recognised them in the state he was in.

He needed it. Now.

Strangely, Bradley did not make a habit of shooting heroin. He enjoyed the relaxing effects of the drug a few times a year and only used it when he truly needed to escape reality.

He had tried most drugs at an early age but felt as though he was in control of his drug use, otherwise it got in the way of his business ventures. He constantly proved his inner strength by not letting the drugs take him over. His life had been funded - but not ruled - by illegal drugs for as long as he could remember, and he knew no better. But he did know the importance of money, and wanted to make a lot of it.

Over the last six months Lorraine had been 'keeping him in check'; she had forced him to reduce the risks he took by only dealing to a little over half of his normal clientele. If he had an office, there would be a sign hanging on the door saying: WE ARE NOT TAKING ANY NEW CLIENTS FOR NOW. WE APOLOGISE FOR THE INCONVENIENCE. This, for the time being, made Lorraine much happier. Bradley knew his mates thought he was pussy-whipped, but he didn't mind. He felt his life was on track with Lorraine around. Almost like feeling happy for the first time.

He strode into the neat lounge room and set down the black container. Despite having drunk a full glass of bourbon, Bradley was able to focus on the fact that he was still without fire, essential for cooking heroin. He racked his brain over where he could find a lighter.

Humans prioritise things, and smokers prioritise everything relating to smoking. Smokers may not know how much coffee they have in their house, even if they particularly enjoy coffee, but they will always know where all their tobacco products are hidden or even subconsciously 'forgotten' about around the house.

Bradley knew. He knew that last weekend Lorraine screamed the house down because he had been smoking inside (his own house) again, after she kindly asked (told) him not to. He knew she'd turned the place upside-down and found every cigarette, tobacco product, bong, cone, lighter and rolling paper, and thrown them all in the rubbish.

At the time, he didn't mind. He loved her. He'd never had a woman like her. She cared. She had sass. She had attitude. She was the start-up phase of the permutation that his life required. He enjoyed her strength, her self-respect – it had been a rarity in his past romances. He would do anything for her. And, even though it had been an absolute failure, tonight's deal was what Bradley would describe as a 'step in the right direction'.

None of that helped him cook his heroin though.

Then he remembered the butane stove.

Meanwhile, the draught from the open window

had pushed the flame against the butane canister and Bradley was lucky he'd left the room when the gas bottle detonated. Flames ran up the curtain, spread across the walls and lapped at the ceiling.

Bradley raced to the kitchen, sobering up as he took in the flaming kitchen. His thoughts went to his secret storage place in the kitchen ceiling where he stored his nest egg. The small safe bolted to a ceiling strut required a six-digit code, which only he knew. No drugs, just cash. And at last count he had $22,000 in used notes. This was a substantial amount to Bradley, and under no circumstances could he lose it.

He rushed to the laundry, grabbed the fire extinguisher from the wall, and clumsily doused the burning ceiling. The flames were surging toward the manhole that covered the access to the safe. He sprayed the fire but the small extinguisher seemed to be no match for the flames. He needed to get to that manhole. After another thirty seconds of wetting the ceiling, the flames finally appeared to be submitting.

He fumbled with the extinguisher several times before dropping it to the floor, grabbing a kitchen stool and shoving it under the dripping manhole cover. He then leapt onto the stool and pushed out the manhole cover, reaching for the safe which was another arm's length beyond his fingertips.

The air from his movements fanned the guttering

flame on the wall which crept up the hot, charred window frame and spread over the ceiling.

Bradley was so focused on getting to his money that he heard and felt nothing. With his head inside the ceiling space, tapping the safe code digits as quickly as he could, he was oblivious until the flame whooshed up through the manhole and hit him in the face. He fell off the stool as skin reddened and swelled on his forehead and nose. Fortunately for Bradley, he missed all the bench corners and other objects in the kitchen, but he was knocked out cold when his head hit the tiled floor.

When Bradley came to, the kitchen was fully alight. Each breath he took was searing hot, filling his lungs with smoke and ash.

His head hurt. His face stung. He touched his nose and winced, looking at his fingers and seeing red, wet, sticking skin. He felt dizzy. The room was full of dark smoke and the roof was well alight.

He struggled to his feet, and stared one last time at his nest egg as it went up in flames. It never occurred to him that the contents of the safe would probably survive the fire he had inadvertently created. He fell to his knees, fighting the smoke, and eyed the long hallway ahead, his only chance of escape. Bradley crawled, falling to his stomach, creeping past the four framed prints on the hallway wall; he finally reached the front door. Bradley collapsed as he pulled open the door and breathed in the luscious fresh air.

The keys, still in the door, chinked together, the last thing he heard before he passed out.

22:35 hrs – Princess Alexandra Hospital Mental Health Facility

Syd left Riley and her mother in capable hands at mental health reception. They were under no obligation to stay. It was, in essence, a place for people who wanted someone to chat to, rather than the 'treatment' areas and seclusion rooms which were immediately next door, under heavy surveillance.

The hospital still seemed unreasonably calm for an evening, and Syd felt a little eerie as he strolled down the long, white hallway. The squeaks of his boots echoed. This particular section of the hospital was quite old, most likely steeped in history and, Syd expected, stories of the most eerie and haunting. A tingle down his spine made him pick up his pace as he imagined a scream echoing down the long narrow corridor.

He giggled nervously – he was being silly – but he still increased his speed. When his access pass beeped him into the emergency department, he gave a tiny startled jump.

He swung the door open and could feel his heart rate immediately drop fifteen beats a minute. The sight of emergency department nurses buzzing around was reassuring and the familiar hospital sounds were music to his ears. He smiled at the administration clerk and she smiled back.

'Brrr, it's cold in there,' he said to her.

'Maybe it's all the ghosts,' she said, still smiling.

'I'm gonna pretend you didn't just say that. I think there may actually be ghosts in there you know,' Syd said, faking a scared look. She smiled. 'Are you able to tell me which bed Sebastian Silva is in?'

'Sure,' she licked her lips and, after a few mouse clicks, said, 'he's still in ED awaiting surgery. Bed ten.'

'Thank you, Bronte.'

She looked surprised that Syd knew her name, and maybe embarrassed she didn't know his. 'Have a nice night.' She watched discreetly, maybe interested, as he walked away from her.

As Syd turned the corner to visit Sebastian, he ran into Cameron leaving the tea room munching crisps by the handful. Crisps flew everywhere as the bag tumbled out of his hands. Cam stood stunned, his mouth open, looking at Syd. At exactly the same time, Syd thought he saw Amber's unmistakable red ponytail through the thin curtains further up the busy hallway.

For a second, Syd looked as bewildered as Cam.

'Jeez man, look out where you're goin' would you!' Cam's accent thickened when primitive emotions were stirred.

'Ah shit, sorry mate, I'll get you another one, I … just … want to go and see if …' Syd didn't pay any attention to the crisps, or the floor; mesmerised by the possibility of seeing Amber.

He hurried to bed ten, peered in and saw Sebastian sitting up and alert.

'*Hola amigo.* Do you know when you'll be operated on?' Syd asked. The Argentinian smiled and opened his arms.

'*Hola*! Sydney! Mate! How are you? I do not know yet when will they operate. Hopefully soon, eh?'

'Hey, I'll be back in a minute; I have to go and see someone.'

'No worries man.'

Syd let go of the curtain, and he and Amber

locked eyes as she walked out of the consultants room with her doctor friend Marcia. She hesitated at the doorway as Syd walked towards her smiling.

'Hey! What are you doing here? I thought you were at Marcia's tonight?'

Marcia smiled uncomfortably at Syd and made herself scarce.

'Well … Marcia got a call up, and … her car is at the mechanics … so I drove her in. I thought I'd come and say hello,' she said, twirling her hair.

'Okay, I was just popping through to see a patient from earlier tonight.' Syd swayed back and pointed toward Sebastian's space.

Silence. That silence again. Cogs turning

'How are you feeling about the stabbing?' she said with genuine concern.

'Jeez, news travels fast doesn't it? Well I haven't had that much time to think about it really. Maybe once this nightshift is done I can process it a little. It is sad though.' He looked around, wanting to change the subject. 'I can't believe how few people are here tonight. I've never seen it this qui—'

'Ah! Don't say it!' Amber interrupted. 'Never say it's the Q word, because soon it won't be, and it'll be your fault.'

'Oh, yes. Oops.' Syd covered his mouth jokingly. 'What's it to you? You're not working.'

'I'm doing it for my colleagues, Sydney.'

They both smiled.

'Hey, I'm going to go, we've been here a while now. Comms will be hounding us soon,' he half turned, then added casually, 'I thought I saw you coming out of one of the beds up there …'

'Yeah, I thought Marcia was treating someone in there and I needed to see her before I left.'

'The tib-fib? The Argentinian? Ah, that's cool, you could practise your Spanish with him.'

Amber gave a forced, tight-lipped smile, her head bowed.

'I'm joking, Amber,' said Syd, misreading the body language.

'Okay, so I'm not as good as you at speaking Spanish!'

'Oh god, this is getting boring, Amber. It's not necessary you know.' Syd paused, stepped closer and lowered his voice. 'Is there something wrong? Seriously? On the phone, earlier tonight, didn't you say we needed to talk?' He spoke directly and with no spite.

She looked around, then took his hand and said, 'Come with me.' She led him around a corner and buzzed them both into the clean linen room.

As soon as she shut and locked the door, Amber slammed Syd around against the wall, standing on tiptoes to reach his mouth in a passionate kiss. He could taste chocolate on her lips and smell masses of clean government laundry.

'What the fuck? If we get caught—'

'Be quick then,' she said lasciviously.

Syd caught the look in her eyes – desire, arousal, control – a look he had grown accustomed to seeing in Amber, and one that he knew required prompt attention.

He cupped her face and pressed his other hand against her lower back, pulling her close to him, kissing her deeply. She undid three of his shirt buttons and stroked his body, rubbing her petite fingers through his hair while she ground against his thigh.

He moved his hand down and squeezed her arse, forcing her to grind even harder. He breathed against her cheek and felt her breath in his ear. Syd leaned back against the wall, propping himself up and creating an almost horizontal pole with his thigh, so that Amber could rub herself against him. She kept both her hands inside his shirt, squeezing his muscles and occasionally pulling at his hair.

He could feel her wetness coming through both their pants.

Amber breathed more and more quickly, rubbing and pushing and moaning. Soon she put all her weight on his thigh and fucked harder and faster. Then in one almighty shove she came in a torrent of shuddering and suppressed cries, crawling closer to Syd's body, wanting to be held.

He pulled her close.

'Fuck you're good,' she said.

'Hmm, you did most of the—'

'Shhh.' She hugged him, then grabbed his face and kissed him hard.

'Let's see how quick you can make it,' she said, touching Syd's wet thigh. She unclipped his work belt as if she'd engineered it, then unbuttoned his pants and unzipped his fly. Her fingers crept down his balls, palm pressed firmly against his shaft. He shuddered as she tickled him lightly, feeling her rise with his cock in her dominant left hand. She pushed him back so he was bolt upright against the wall, then she turned, grabbed a hospital blanket, and threw it on the ground between his legs. It took him a moment to understand, then he struggled to hide a huge grin.

She grabbed his face and kissed him hard, jerking his cock.

'Come,' she said in the most demanding tone she'd ever used. Then she dropped to her knees, never missing a stroke, and licked the length of his shaft before closing her lips around his cock. It's not that he was huge; it was just that she was never able to deep throat. Sydney stood looking down on her beautiful red ponytail bouncing back and forth while she increased her grip.

He could feel her tongue curl around the underside of his cock, moving like they were made for each other.

He was close.

She could sense it as he grew that last bit.

She took his cock out of her mouth, jerking it hard and sliding up and down the full wet length, her fingers pushed up behind his balls.

She looked up at him. 'Come, Sydney.'

The tingling started in his feet then moved up his legs to his groin, then exploded into her mouth, while she pulled faster and faster. The sensation continued up his spine, standing all his hair on end, and up to his head; it was an addictive high.

He tried to muffle his cry, but it was still audible outside the room, after which he settled.

'Is *that* what you wanted to talk about? Amber, you are a stick of dynamite,' Syd said lovingly, trying to control his shuddering.

Amber stood up, looked him in the eyes, and swallowed purposefully.

'*You're* the stick of dynamite,' she replied in a cheeky, girlish tone, 'but we really should get out of here in case someone heard you explode.'

One year earlier – Riley

Riley lay on her bed reading.

'Riley, quick, get in the car please, we are leaving now.' Karen's volume was ratcheting up as she hammered on Riley's bedroom door.

The girl moved across the room to her door and opened it quickly, as though trying to surprise her mother. She had moved on though, and Riley heard the clinking of cutlery and dishes. She strolled unhurriedly further down the hallway.

Karen was bending over the dishwasher, transferring clean dishes to a cupboard in a robotic movement.

'What are you doing, Mum?' Riley asked.

'Quickly, Riley, we're leaving as of five minutes

ago.'

'Where are we going?' Riley asked coolly.

'You know where. To the airport to pick up your father.'

There were no more dishes to be unpacked but Karen continued to tidy as though possessed.

'Oh, do I really need to come with you?'

'Of course, Riley. You haven't seen your father in over two weeks. Think about how happy he'll be to see you.'

'Yeah, he'll see me when he gets home too, you know,' said Riley, 'I'm in my pyjamas Mum. And it's *nine-thirty*. There's no way I'm leaving this house tonight. No way.' Riley leaned against the door jamb and crossed her arms.

'Please Riley, don't upset me, I asked nicely. Now please go and get in the car.'

'Why would you leave it till the last minute to tell me about this? Seriously.'

'I told you about it this morning Riley,' Karen said pleasantly.

'I haven't seen you since *last night*, Mum. What are you talking about?' Riley began to raise her voice.

Karen wiped down the sink, which was already spotless, and turned to Riley, who still stood with her arms crossed. Karen took two bounding steps towards her and yelled, 'Your father would really like to see you, Riley. *At the fucking airport!* Now get in the fucking car!' She brandished the dishcloth in Riley's face as though it was a weapon.

As usual, Karen's driving was anything but safe as she headed for the airport to collect her husband Jerry. Neither mother nor daughter noticed the silence between them as Riley gripped her seat and Karen halved the time it would normally take to drive that distance. She drove erratically and dangerously, and Riley, yet to hold even a learner's permit, silently questioned how her mother ever got her licence.

Riley dared not speak but wondered if her mother was doing this speed racer challenge for any particular reason. Maybe she only remembered her husband at the last minute, but was that likely three times in three months? Surely not.

Their timing couldn't have been any more perfect; Karen pulled up just as Jerry walked into the airport pickup bay. She popped the boot and hurried to meet him with wide arms and a huge smile. 'Darling! How was your flight?'

Jerry carefully placed the suitcase in the boot and closed the lid. Karen hugged him tightly, almost desperately, but he spun out of the embrace without a word.

'Is everything okay, darling?' Karen asked as Riley jumped out of the front passenger seat and opened the back door.

Jerry's eyes lit up. 'Riley! Honey! How was

school?' He turned his back to Karen and hugged Riley.

Karen seemed to shrink as her shoulders slumped.

'Hey Dad,' said Riley, 'I'm, like, in my pyjamas you know. Let me hide!'

22:40 hrs – Bravo 989

The Mercedes Sprinter drove through the slowly diminishing traffic, returning to the station once again.

'So are you all right about tonight so far, son?' Cameron said as he drove.

'Yeah … it's really only been the stabbing that's been hectic,' Syd replied. 'Did you see a lot of stabbings when you were in Glasgow?'

'Aye … trauma was a pretty regular thing we had to manage.' Cam paused as he slowed for a red light. 'And I remember when I was new to it. It stressed me out a fair bit at the start. I was young, freshly married, and Claire was pregnant. It was a different world for me. And work consisted of trying to keep these *bealin'* crazy patients alive after they had stabbed or shot each other or just—'

'What's *bealin'*?' Syd interrupted.

'Ah. Sorry son. *Bealin'* means fookin' angry. Crazy angry.'

Syd watched Cam as he revved and drove again.

'We didn't really talk about our feelings in those days neither,' he continued. 'We'd see all this bad shite happen and be right in the middle of it and management wouldn't care, we were always expected to keep a stiff upper lip. The attitude was, *if we couldn't handle it, we could get out of it.*' Cam took a deep breath. 'And then management finally clicked onto the paramedics' suicide rate being abnormally high, and thought, *well, this statistic doesn't look very good on our spreadsheet does it?*' Cam used a dopey voice.

'Ah huh,' Syd said, letting Cam know that he was still there, listening.

The dopey voice continued. '*So, we might see if we can get some other strategy to keep these paramedics from going nuts.*'

'And that's when they hired counsellors or something?'

'Aye, son, something like that. It was only really coming into effect when I left Scotland and it was in full swing here already. I'd been in the job for ten years by that stage.'

'And probably would've seen pretty much

everything,' said Syd, 'and dealt with it too.'

'Yeah. I suppose. Ah, not really though son. You've never seen everything. Don't think that you have; it'll make you complacent. But the bad shite I did see, I wasn't by myself. This is what I'm sayin' to you son. I was lucky 'cause Claire knew me well and made me talk to her.' He looked over at Syd with a quick deep stare, 'and I think that's what kept me sane.'

Syd nodded, sensing Cam was maybe feeling emotional.

'Anyway, son, whatever happened to me has happened. You, on the other hand, need to look after yourself and know what to look out for.'

Syd feigned a smile.

'I'm serious son. Don't fook around with this. It'll come back to bite you.'

'So, if I feel stressed out, or upset about a job, I go and talk to someone, right?'

The radio interrupted abruptly, 'Bravo 989?'

'That's exactly right,' Cam said as Syd reached for the handpiece. Cam raised his hand signalling for Syd to wait. 'And don't be scared to talk to me either, son.' Syd nodded and reached again, then realized Cam was looking for a stronger reassurance.

'I won't Cam. Thank you,' Syd said, looking straight at Cam, then turned his attention to the volume dial and increased it slightly.

'Bravo 989,' he said.

'Bravo 989 what's you location?'

'Bravo 989 we are currently, ah …?' Syd, still thinking about their conversation, forgot to release the UHF microphone button. 'Where the fuck are—'

'On Old Cleveland Road, just coming into Carina,' Cameron cut in. Syd hastily repeated the information, feeling inept because the *whole service* had just heard him swear on the radio.

'Bravo 989, you are the closest and primary unit to an urgent call from QFRS who are on scene at 173 Randwick Road, Carina. They have a male patient, unconscious, breathing, who was found on location. Reported to have severe facial burns and breathing difficulty. The location is fully ablaze but the patient is now clear of the fire,' said the droning female voice.

'On case,' Syd said as he finished tapping the address into the GPS. 'GPS says we're three minutes away, comms.'

Cameron flicked the switches for bright lights and sirens, and sped off.

'I haven't done airway burns yet Cam,' Syd said nervously as Cam slid the ambulance around a clear corner.

'Again, mate, hopefully ICPs will be there to intubate if need be. Otherwise, it's just what?' Cam asked, testing Syd.

'Thorough primary assessment, airway

management, and later pain management. Lots of oxygen if carbon monoxide intake. Active cooling twenty minutes if burns.'

'They say to estimate burnt surface area too,' said Cam.

The predicted three minutes was in fact one due to Cam's careful but speedy driving.

The scene was tight, space was at a premium, and Cam nearly nudged a second fire truck as it entered at the same time. The ambulance parked right next to the patient, who lay on the dirty lawn of the house next door. The fire fighters continued to spray powerful jets of water at the house, which was fully ablaze.

'Grab the oxygen and the airways,' Cam instructed as he took a pair of trauma shears from the dash, climbed out and walked the short distance to the patient. Syd did as instructed and went to Cam, who had already cut the patient's tracksuit top off and was feeling for a carotid pulse.

'Put the O_2 on, I can't really see shite out here. Grab the stretcher and scoop and we'll work in the truck. He's got a good pulse and is breathing shallow.'

Again Sydney followed instructions and connected a plastic mask to the small oxygen cylinder, turned it onto maximum and gently put the mask on the patient's face, as he noted the glistening burns.

As he turned to retrieve the stretcher, he heard Cam say loudly, 'Can you hear me sir? Open your eyes!' Syd felt a millisecond of amusement mixed with adrenaline as he noted Cameron's accent had grown thicker through urgency and concern.

Sydney promptly returned to the patient with the stretcher, then split the scoop in two and placed one half next to the patient, whose eyes had begun to flutter.

Cameron grabbed the other half and clacked them together, forming a hard, handled board beneath the patient. Cameron asked a nearby fire fighter, who seemed to not be fighting fire at the time, to help lift the scooped patient onto the stretcher and into the ambulance. The burly fireman was more than happy to help.

Cameron jumped into the ambulance and dropped into the rear-facing seat, used to supervise a patient's airway, as Sonia the ICP arrived. She poked her head in and asked with her characteristic positive energy, 'So what have we got guys?'

'Hey Sonia, we've got a male of unknown age, facial burns, not sure about the airway yet, it was difficult to see, but breathing shallow at 30, pulse around 130, bounding, haven't checked anything else yet,' said Cam.

'Great, Cameron. I might just sit there in case I have to tube him.' Sonia spoke with purpose but without arrogance. She swapped Cam in the airway seat and turned to Syd, who stood between the open rear doors of the ambulance, 'Do you mind asking around to make sure there's no other patients please Sydney? Also find out if the firies are going in with breathing apparatus. We'll need another crew out here if they are.'

Syd nodded and went to find the answers from a senior fire fighter. He found himself moving briskly but calmly, completely focused. It felt good. He spoke clearly and listened closely.

The building had been checked and cleared for other patients, and the fire fighters had used breathing apparatuses.

Soon Syd had returned to the back of the ambulance and reported to Sonia, Cameron, and the now near-naked patient.

Sonia listened and said, 'Can you tell comms to send another—'

'I've already phoned CDS for one. They'll be about six minutes,' Syd interrupted, pleased to know that another ambulance would be needed, and that he had organised it.

'Great, Sydney,' Sonia smiled, 'so, we've tubed our patient and given Midazolam and Morphine to keep him settled. He is breathing on his own but due to the facial burns there may be some airway compromise so we're just staying on the safe side.' Sonia spoke as though she was checking off a list in her mind, rather than looking for confirmation from

Cam or Syd. With Cam's assistance, she had put a tube down the patient's throat and into the trachea, to secure the airway, in case the patient had breathed in fire, causing his airway to swell.

'The whole face, frontal scalp and left temporal have superficial dermal burns, he's on 15 litres O_2, spO_2 reading 100 per cent, resp rate at 24, tachycardic at 120, everything else is A-OK-ish. He has those strange long, wide lumps on the stomach and chest, but I don't think they are too much to worry about yet. Let's get a move on Sydney, code one to the PA. Have you done much code one driving?'

'A couple of times with the crew in the back,' said Syd.

'Without wanting to be patronising, Sydney, just think of us as goldfish back here – if you drive crazily we'll spill out of our bowl, okay?' She smiled again, a striking, genuine smile. Syd felt a shiver, smiled back, nodded and shut the door.

Aside from Sonia's phone call to the ED, so they could prepare for the patient, the ten-minute drive was uneventful. Sonia and Cameron worked efficiently together, and Sydney's driving was so careful, he thought he must have had one eye on the road and one on the rear-view mirror the entire time, being sure not to tip the bowl too much.

23:05 hrs – Princess Alexandra Hospital Emergency Department

Sonia took care of the hospital handover, relaying the relevant information she found in Bradley's wallet to police, who had followed the ambulance to hospital.

Doctor Das smiled at Sonia and Syd as his team went to work on the unconscious Bradley, prodding, poking, testing.

The buzz of the ED felt good to Syd. He liked how everyone knew their role and how to communicate all necessary information. He was impressed every time. He rolled the empty stretcher out of the ED and faced the ward beds. His eyes stung slightly, a common feeling during night shift, although it didn't usually take hold until early morning. He blinked as he looked at cubicle ten, Sebastian's.

He blinked again - this time in disbelief - as Amber hurried out through the curtain. Suddenly sickness stirred in his stomach and he felt a deep ache in his chest. He began to breathe quickly as he thought about Amber's recent behaviour.

Life is too short.

She breezed away from him, ponytail bouncing. His mind was filled with jealousy, love and trust, all awash with intense confusion. He felt dizzy but he had to ask her what was going on.

He steamed up to Sebastian's cubicle as Amber disappeared into the consultants room about fifteen metres away. He glanced inside and saw Sebastian as before, sitting up, awake and alert.

'Hey! Sydney! Mate! You still here?'

'Hey Sebastian,' Syd said mournfully. 'Hey that nurse who just walked out of here, is she taking good care of you?'

And without a moment's hesitation, Sebastian replied, 'Ah, she sure is Sydney mate! That is my girlfriend, the one I was telling you about, remember?' Sebastian smiled innocently.

'Oh, fuck.'

Life is too short.

'I did not even know she was working at this hospital lately, she is an agency nurse and can ...' Sebastian continued.

The sickness grew in Syd's stomach; he could feel it rising up. His face felt red and hot. He was angry; he was sad; he wanted to release a flood of tears and simultaneously punch Sebastian's face till it bled. He moved behind the curtain.

'Hey, Sydney? Mate?' Sebastian said gently.

Syd breathed in deeply, trying to calm himself. He clutched at the curtain, then, aware of the nearby medical professionals, some of whom he knew, tried to regain his composure. He looked at the consultants room. He had to know. He had to ask her. He had to confront her. *His* girlfriend? *Whose* girlfriend? *What the fuck?*

Just the thought of the words made his anger boil up. He wanted to yell. He wanted to hit something. He wanted to unleash all the crazy confusion that now filled his stupid trusting head. He stormed the fifteen paces to the consultants' room, struggling to appear calm, knowing that some of the staff would notice for sure.

Where could he confront her? Right here? At work? *In front of everyone?*

No. He would contain his feelings and see if Amber would talk somewhere private.

As Syd raised his knuckles to knock on the door, it was pulled open and three doctors moved swiftly past him. He entered the room and saw Amber and two other uniformed nurses chatting. Amber noticed Sydney immediately and registered his body language. She sent him a look of big-eyed innocence, and then got up to walk to him.

Syd knew he must have looked intense, possibly even a mess – red in the face, fists clenched – so he purposefully slowed his breathing. He tried to control himself, but erupted, loudly enough for the whole room to hear him clearly: 'What the fuck is going on Amber?'

She stopped about three steps from him. The chatting nurses fell silent as one of them said in a loud warning tone, 'Are you okay, Amber?'

She looked Syd in the eye, as a tear forced its way out and ran down his cheek.

'Thanks, I'll be okay.' Amber took another step and asked, 'Can we go somewhere to talk?'

Syd opened both hands and said, 'You lead.'

Amber walked slowly past him while watching his eyes, and then out the door, leading him to the empty family room, where family members could wait while critical care was provided to their injured or dying loved ones. Syd thought it fitting: this was going to be a critical conversation, one that might result in the death of their relationship.

Amber closed the door behind Syd. The windowless room was small, but enough for two cheap double-seater couches, a bench, sink, and mini fridge. He felt claustrophobic; he wanted to jump out; he wanted to be in a plane.

'I told you we needed to talk,' Amber said, 'but I didn't want it to be like this.'

'What the fuck are you talking about, Amber? He says *you're his girlfriend!* My patient from tonight!' Syd stood with his left calf muscle pushing against the couch, a subconscious reminder to himself not to move.

Amber pouted at Syd then looked down.

'The Argentinian!'

'I know, I know,' she sighed, 'I know the Argentinian.' She stared at the floor in silence. She took a deep breath. 'We've been together since he arrived in Australia nine months ago.'

Syd's shoulders dropped as he let out a purposeful sigh.

More silence.

'The *whole time we've been together*? What? *Why?*' Syd spoke in a less aggressive tone, as though a weight had lifted from his mind now that Amber had at least admitted her disloyalty.

'I don't know why, Sydney. I have no real answer. I care for you both very deeply.' She wouldn't meet his eye.

'Holy fuck. I can't believe you're going to try that angle. Fucking bullshit Amber! Rather than actually admitting you're addicted to the attention? Or something like that? And the sex too, no doubt? God

I can't imagine how that guy fucks you.' Syd repulsed himself with his own words. 'Fuck! What is wrong with you? I fucking love you!'

Amber glanced up at Syd. 'And I … love you too, Sydney. I love hearing you say it actually. I *really do* love you,' she said, stepping closer, slowly, dramatically, as though she was now convinced. He pushed back on the couch and they both paused.

'You *can't* love me Amber. You've been with another person the *whole four months* we've been together!' Syd continued to fight back the tears and to contain his apoplectic mood.

'I do, Sydney, love … *you*,' she said sexily and swayed in even closer. 'And after all the help we have given each other? We can't lose that. You helping me open up the way you have, emotionally I mean, and I've helped you with your studies and chatting about jobs, and you know we both love being together … Sydney?'

Syd glared at Amber, noticing how gorgeous she was when she creased her eyebrows that little bit. He wondered if he could forget about what he now knew, and continue to feel the love and passion he had felt so wholeheartedly for this woman.

'I can keep helping you, you know, I won't stop Sydney. I love helping and teaching and we've learnt so much together, you know? We've had a great time, you know we have. And the sex Sydney … oh the sex.' Amber spoke girlishly. 'I know now I love *you* Sydney.'

'I think I may be going crazy listening to you say this stuff. This is not the Amber I know,' Syd said. 'Even though this is all very raw, I still have the sense to know you've cheated on me all that time we were *helping* each other. I'm not thanking you for that, in fact, fuck this—'

'Sydney, please, I'm really sorry,' she said calmly. 'I do, really love you.'

'What on earth did you want to *talk to me about? When you didn't want it to be like this*? "Ah yes, Sydney, honey, we need to talk. Um, I've been fucking another bloke the entire time we've been together. Just thought I'd tell you, but that's okay isn't it? Because we're so close and we have so much in common. Just letting you know honey ..."' Syd barked.

'I wanted to tell you, Sydney. I felt terrible earlier tonight.'

'Wait. Hold the fuck on.' Syd paused. There was no sound. '*I'm* the other bloke aren't I? Not him. He's the *actual* boyfriend.'

'Sydney I have made a mistake—'

'You've been with him for nine months, Amber! *Nine months*. Are you fucking nuts? I hope you *are* nuts, then you will *at least* have a diagnosis, rather than simply being an attention-seeking dick-hungry lier.' Syd's temporal vein was visible.

She narrowed her eyes and pressed her lips

together. Then, as though she'd flicked a switch, she straightened up, looked Syd straight in the eye and said, 'I'm sorry. It will never happen again. I love you.'

'What? No. You can't. You can't say that. Do you go out to dinner with the Argentinian, or on adventures, or walks, or just have sex, or … ah … I don't know, what do you do?' Syd spat.

As Amber drew breath to reply, he cut in, 'Actually it doesn't even matter what you *think* the answer is. Fuck this, I'm outta here.'

Amber leapt forward and wrapped her arms around him hard. 'I'm *so sorry* Sydney,' she said, 'I only want *you*.'

Syd's body stiffened, repelled by her touch. He was dumbfounded. 'Amber. You are obsessed with the attention. Now get the fuck off me. I have to think.'

She released him and turned her back, head bent. He could hear her forcing out the sobs as he opened the door. He felt he should say something more to her, but could think of nothing remotely suitable.

He walked out and past bed ten, trying not to wonder if Sebastian knew too. He thought infidelity disgraceful, and felt ashamed and embarrassed that this was their story. He felt completely alone, but told himself firmly that not everyone was out to get him. Although he had only met Sebastian tonight, *as a patient*, he wondered if it was all 'just meant to be'. He hoped that it was; that this had happened for a reason and that better things would come in time. His attempt at positive thinking didn't stop a heaped handful of salt being rubbed into the wound though.

He felt the familiar vibration of the pager on his hip and clicked the button:

CODE 2B – 25A1 – NON-SUICIDAL AND ALERT – 455 TOTTENHAM STREET – WOOLLOONGABBA

He walked the wrong way, numb, unable to concentrate on the simple things. Without really paying any attention, he was heading toward the desk where Bronte sat. As soon as she glanced up from her desk and shot him a smile, he realised where he was, and stood blinking at her like a deer in the headlights.

'Are you going back to see the ghosts again?'

Syd wiped his palms on his pants, looking like he should be in one of the mental health seclusion rooms, then turned and shuffled away. Bronte looked puzzled.

Syd's circling thoughts paralysed him. Maybe *Sebastian* had no idea? Maybe *Amber* had plotted this the entire time? To have *two* boyfriends, *two* partners, *two lovers*? Maybe he *and* she both knew and didn't care? But she knew what? She knew everything didn't she?

Life. It is way too short.

Ten years earlier – Sonia

A whirly-whirly funnelled the dust and moved erratically across the ground, passing over two huts and across a football field, which was completely devoid of grass, increasing in size as it approached the far goal. The fifteen barefoot Kenyan children who played there ignored the dust devil completely, focusing on their ratty football as they passed and scored.

These were the happiest kids she had ever seen.

Sonia was the fifteen-year-old daughter of missionary parents. She had travelled with them through Central America, the Middle East, and Africa: in fact this was the fourth African country in two years. She was home-schooled by her parents although it was rare for her to learn anything she hadn't already found in a textbook. Her parents were simple and caring people. Christians to their core, they believed that if they spread the Gospel far enough, they would be amongst the anointed and in the very best position to meet Jesus when He returned. They taught the Bible with an intensity bordering on ferocity to both young and old in the Third World countries they visited. They believed that Africa had to change, and what they taught was the start of that change. There was always a school or church needing to be built, so their semi-professional building skills were continually useful. The ministry provided food, clothing and shelter to those who took the Lord into their hearts and spread God's love; predictably, that was almost every soul in the villages where they worked.

Sonia walked towards the main part of the town, Turbi, which she could see in the distance. The whirly-whirly filled her eyes with dust, and she rubbed them clear once the vortex had finished with her. It was quite a strong whirly, and Sonia felt as though it had lifted her somewhat. She smiled as she continued towards town, where, today, she would be teaching her loving primary-school students her favourite subject: science.

She loved the children's joy in learning, the wonderful innocence of their minds, and was humbled by the absolute respect they showed, even though she was a fifteen-year-old, unqualified teacher. Sonia loved her students.

The whirly continued, following the main dirt road towards town and passing a large yard of camels. As the sheds became shops and the road began to narrow, the whirly started to thin. It had lost its drive. It faded from the top, and before long, it was nothing but a breath of red dust, brushing the heels of a member of the Borana tribe, who stood looking over a village block, holding a machete in each hand.

His head was wrapped in a striped rag of blue, orange and green, his eyes were bloodshot, his torso swathed in sky-blue cloth, and behind him stood thirty warriors in similar dress, armed with similar weapons.

Suddenly, the small army of Borana tribesmen spread out and rushed toward the homes and shops. Sonia heard the yells and taunts, the screams. She was well aware of the tensions between the two local tribes, having heard about their bloody history from her primary students who lived in fear of the Borana. She panicked. Despite all the advice her parents had given her about staying clear of tribal problems, she thought of her students. What could she do? She had no idea. So she ran. She ran as fast as she could towards the bloodcurdling screams.

The closer she got, the more clearly she could see and the louder the sounds of attack and retreat were. By the time she reached the shops, the Borana had moved on, retreating south, back to their own village.

Amongst the mental images of the massacre, which Sonia would never be able to forget, were those of twenty-two of her primary school class, and both her parents.

She wept for weeks.

23:40 hrs – Princess Alexandra Hospital Emergency Department

Syd's mind dizzied as he walked through the ED and saw Cam and Sonia in the write-up room completing paperwork. He tried to avoid being seen as he strolled past the door, which made his presence more obvious, and pressed the green exit button for the automatic doors. The crisp air hit his face and arms, raising goosebumps, and at the same time he heard the write-up room door open behind him. He hesitated.

'Hi Sydney, are you okay?' Sonia said.

He opened his eyes wide and blinked, before he

turned and said, 'Hey Sonia, yeah, all okay, thanks. How much longer are you guys going to be? We just got another job.'

His face still felt red, and he could feel the drying tears on his cheeks, but he didn't touch them.

'Well, you don't look okay. We have to look after you students,' she said, smiling. 'I'm happy to chat about it if you like?'

The automatic doors closed.

'Aah, no, it's okay, it's not work-related stuff. Work's fine,' he said unconvincingly, and reached out and hit the green button again.

'Look, Sydney, it's been a big night for you guys, Cameron was telling me.' Sonia came right up to Syd and gently grasped his elbow. Her hand was warm. 'Especially with that stabbing, *and the wife,* and now this fire. If you have any concerns and don't talk about it—'

'Jeez I haven't had time to think about all that,' Syd cut in, recalling the events of the night's work, 'Maybe it's just better not to think about it right now.' Syd looked into Sonia's kind eyes, then turned away. 'I've just been having some relationship issues with my girlfriend, that's all. And they're being addressed tonight, *here* and *now.*'

The doors closed.

'Oh that's rough. Is she a patient or staff?'

'You wouldn't believe me if I told you.'

'Try me. I've had my fair share of relationship

issues.'

'And I've only *just now* found out, as in, two fuckin' minutes ago. I'm probably not making any sense anyway,' Syd caught himself, realising he was nervous.

Sonia moved even closer. 'Okay. Okay. No problems Sydney. I don't want to push you at all. But I am more than happy to chat about whatever you like, whenever you like. Okay?' Her blue eyes locked onto his. He felt instantly aroused, realised it, and then dismissed it by reaching for the green button once more.

'Well it looks like we've got another one, son.' Cam's booming voice broke open the moment. 'Let's get a move on, and save this muppet from bringing any joy to the world.' The two of them shot him an anxious look, and he understood Sonia's much better than Syd's. 'Is everything all right?'

'Hey Cam, Syd's just having a crappy time at the moment. Maybe you could do patient care for this one?' Sonia suggested.

Syd looked away.

'For sure, Sonia. No problems, lad. Hey I've gotta do some of the work haven't I?' Cam said with a grin. 'Sonia, how are you gonna get your car?'

'It's all good, I'll organise someone to drive me back there to pick it up,' said Sonia, turning back to Syd and giving him a heartfelt smile.

23:50 hrs – Bravo 989

Syd drove the ambulance out of the hospital grounds, under the overpass, and one block further then told comms they were 'on scene'.

'Do you want me to bring anything in?'

'Just the de-fib mate,' Cam said as they both left the vehicle. Across the road was a small shopping centre, and although everything was closed, the colourful neon of a typical takeaway store lit up the street.

Four flights of stairs later, the two paramedics found the unit number, and Cam gave a loud, solid double knock on the door. No reply.

Cam knocked again and called, 'Hello? Ambulance,' to which he heard a faint voice inside the unit say, 'Come in, it's unlocked.'

As Cam pushed the door open, they were hit in the face by a pungent stench. Cam stopped and turned, still holding the handle, and Syd slammed into him, following too close behind with other things on his mind.

'Watch it mate,' said Cam, then whispered, 'and take a deep breath.'

The unit was cluttered and slovenly – it was as though Syd and Cam had been teleported into another world, a world where cleanliness and organisation didn't matter, and where simple hygiene was outlawed. The air was thick like exhaust and stank of decaying food and flatulence.

After tripping over litter strewn around the doorway, the two paramedics scanned the lounge room, as if preparing to set sail on a journey into the unknown. An entire corner was dedicated to empty pizza boxes and fast food containers, which were not stacked but thrown carelessly into a pile. Nearby was a similar-sized-pile of newspapers, some opened, some still rolled in plastic wrap. On the other side of the room, near the bedroom door, clothing was piled up in no noticeable order almost to the ceiling.

All available floor space was covered in layers of junk, apart from a narrow path that led, roughly, from the front door to the dark green recliner chair in the middle of the lounge room, then on to the kitchenette and the bedroom. Not a single scrap of carpet or flooring was visible.

The stink of the unit was inescapable. Both paramedics breathed through their mouths, and Syd felt ill, sure he could taste it.

On the dark green recliner chair sat a woman with both arms propped on the armrests and her feet only just reaching the floor. She was morbidly obese and seemed to spill over the chair on which she sat. Her skin was clear and pale, her hair dark and oily, and she wore a dirty green T-shirt with blue tracksuit pants that ended at her knees.

Cam led the way into the urban rubbish jungle.

'Hello,' he said, 'I'm Cameron, what's your name?'

The woman on the recliner didn't move.

'Danielle,' she said.

'Hi Danielle, that's Sydney behind me there. What seems to be the problem this morning?'

'Oh well, I dunno, I think it's the depression. I just need some help. Someone to review me,' she replied breathlessly, rushing her words. Syd instantly thought her voice reminded him of pencil sharpenings: woody and delicate, but jagged, and ready to crumble if squeezed too hard.

'What do you mean you think it's the depression? What's *it*?' said Cam patiently, before turning to Syd and asking him to get a full set of vitals from their new patient.

Syd stood behind Cam, with no room to move. 'Yep, no problem. Just move to your left a bit Cam,' Syd said quietly. He attempted to step around Cam in a kind of 'straddle', as well as keep his feet on the path, but the weight of the defibrillator caused him to overbalance. He grabbed at Cam's arm as he fell backwards, panicking as though he were falling - in what felt like slow motion - into a great canyon ... lined with fire and filled with cannibals.

Syd crashed onto the pizza box pyramid, de-fib still in hand. He jumped up, ripping at an opened pizza box that was stuck to the side of his face. 'Argh fuck!' he said with disgust. 'Oh yuck, what the—'

Cam erupted in laughter.

'Jesus, why do you keep all your rubbish inside?' Syd said.

Danielle bowed her head. 'I'm sorry. I know. I haven't had a chance to clean for a while.'

Cam stopped laughing.

'A while?' said Syd. 'More like an etern—' He paused and gathered himself as he looked down at the enormous sedentary shape on the green recliner. He brushed himself off, 'Oh well, no harm done.'

Danielle forced a smile.

'You all right mate?' Cam managed to ask, deadpan.

'Good,' said Syd, still pissed.

Cam turned back to their patient. 'So, Danielle,

you were telling me what *it* is?'

Danielle paused, still watching Syd.

'Well, I suppose *it* is just that I get down. Upset. Lonely. I don't know what else to say about it really.'

'What's your medical history, Danielle?' Cam asked, as Syd exchanged the regular blood pressure cuff for the super-sized one.

'I've had depression for three years now. I lost my job because of it. I've got diabetes and high blood pressure, but I take medication for that … ah … and osteoarthritis … that's about it I think.'

'And your medications?'

'They're over there, stacked next to the fridge,' she said, pointing to the kitchenette.

'To save us the danger of exploring this trip hazardous area,' Cam said, 'is there any chance you know them off the top of your head?'

'Amlodipine, Diabex XR, Sertraline, oh and also Lipitor, I've got high cholesterol too. Sorry, forgot about that.'

Syd had gathered Danielle's vital signs, written them down and passed them to Cam.

'Well Danielle, everything here looks to be reasonably normal,' he said.

'I'm really sorry about the mess. It's terrible I know,' she said, her eyes flicking between Cam and Syd. Syd gave her a sweet look somewhere between empathy and mild loathing.

'That's okay, Danielle. Now, have you got any further concerns?' Cam asked.

Danielle looked over her left shoulder, peering at the recycling pile. At least she's recycling, Syd thought. This was the first time she had moved since the paramedics arrived.

'We are absolutely not movin' that downstairs for you,' Cam joked. Syd chuckled, waiting for Danielle to get the gag.

'No, I was just hoping one of you could have a look around for my little cat. I haven't seen her in two days, and I don't know why she wouldn't have showed.'

'Can the cat get outside?' Syd asked.

'Yes, yes, the bedroom window is always open to the balcony. She can jump down to the street from there. She's an adventurer, that little cat.'

'Eh, yeah, okay, I'll go have a look,' said Cam unenthusiastically as he picked his way past Syd and Danielle and followed the path towards the bedroom.

'What exactly should I look for? If he can come and go and he's not here now, what signs will I look for?' Cam said, still plotting his course.

'He's a she. Her name is Minty. And for all I know she *could* be asleep on my bed in there. Thank you *so much*,' Danielle spoke with a hopeless ache in her voice, one that Syd guessed was not just troubled, but also desperately lonely.

'I felt so bad. A few days ago, she was circling my legs and I couldn't really tell. Then I heard her purring so I fed her, and I haven't seen her since,' she said to Syd.

'You couldn't tell she was circling your legs? While you were sitting there?' Syd asked.

'Well I heard her purring, that's how I knew,' Danielle replied.

'Yes I understand, but could you feel her touching your legs?'

'Hmm, not really, only on one side – this side,' she said, raising her left hand as though shooing a fly from her fingertip.

'Can you normally feel your legs?'

'Yes, of course I can.'

'Can you feel them now?'

'Of course I can.'

'Do you mind wiggling all your toes then?'

Syd looked down at the long, dirty yellow toenails at the end of Danielle's fat and poorly perfused legs. Both ankles were red, swollen and scattered with tiny dark veins.

Five toes wiggled. The other five did not.

'So, Danielle, are you trying to wiggle those toes on your left?'

'They're moving aren't they?' she said in all seriousness.

'No, they are not. Why don't you move forward a bit and have a look?'

She gazed up at him with worried eyes.

'Can you give me a nice big smile?' Syd said before Danielle even tried to move.

'Is this a test?' she asked.

'It sure is.' Although it was barely noticeable, her smile wasn't equal on both sides. Syd had to tell her twice to keep holding the smile as he looked closely at her well-cushioned face.

'Can you lift your arms above your head Danielle?'

'Of course I can.'

'Well, would you mind doing it?'

She concentrated, pulled a strained face, and lifted her right arm to eye level. Her left arm didn't move. 'I swear I'm telling that arm to move.'

Syd stepped forward and placed his hands in hers, 'Okay now, squeeze my hands as hard as you can.'

Right grip: strong; left: weak.

He then placed his hands on the tops of her meaty knees and said, 'Now push each leg up towards the ceiling.'

Danielle pushed her right leg up a little, but her left leg didn't move. 'You are trying with that left one, right?'

'Right. The left one.'

Cam had returned and stood near Danielle's chair, watching Syd's assessment.

Syd produced a biro and circled it under

Danielle's right and left feet, asking each time if she could feel it, and once again asking after he hadn't circled the biro.

She could not feel most of her left side.

Syd looked up at Cam, 'How much of that did you hear, Cam?'

'Most of it, mate. What you thinkin'?'

'TIA probably, but with her obvious level of inactivity it's hard to know.'

'Treat what you see, son.'

'But we don't do anything for a TIA,' said Syd, before asking, 'do we?'

'What's TIA?' Danielle cut in as the two rudely spoke over her.

'Sorry Danielle,' said Syd, 'a TIA is a Transient Ischemic Attack, or mini-stroke. That means that within the last twenty-four hours, you may have had a blockage to the blood flow to a part of your brain, which may be causing this left-sided weakness.'

'Danielle,' Cam chirped, 'I couldn't find the cat, I'm sure he'll— ah, *she'll* be back soon. For now, though, we gotta take you to hospital. The sooner they can look at your brain the sooner they'll start treatment.' He looked at Syd, 'Mate, do you wanna stay here? I'll race down and throw the drug kit up so you can cannulate for me. Then I'll get the stair chair and organise another crew to help us outta here and down those stairs.'

'Yep, no worries,' said Syd, still crouching at Danielle's portly feet.

'Danielle, is there any other way out of this building besides those stairs?' Cam asked.

'No, there isn't. I'm really sorry you guys.'

Cam followed the path back to the front door while Syd went about gathering more information from the defibrillator.

'So how long have you been with the ambulance?' Danielle asked.

'About nine months,' said Syd, smiling.

'You must like it huh? I can tell you like it.'

'I do. I do like it. It's the first job where I can actually help people who need it, plus there's the surprise element too – you never know what's going to happen each shift, and all that.'

'I'm sorry; I know I probably don't need you guys here. I was just down and—'

'Danielle, if you *are* having a TIA – a mini-stroke – it is absolutely essential that we get you seen. They may be able to help, they may not, it all depends on the onset time of your symptoms.'

'I didn't even call for that. I've just been so sad, so lonely,' she said miserably.

'Well that's no good, but we are going to focus on the possibility of the TIA for now, okay, not so much on the depression. I'm not dismissing it, but that's what we have to deal with right now.'

Cam could be heard stomping up the last flight of

stairs. He followed the path and handed the drug kit to Syd. 'All okay? No changes?' he asked.

'We're just here chatting,' said Syd.

'Oh great,' Cam said, wiping his brow. 'Now Danielle, I need you to think of the time when everything with you was good, as in, you could feel both of your legs and move normally … before you had any motor deficit at all. Tell me when that was, okay?'

'Okay, well, I'm not sure,' she said.

'Well, have a think about it and I'll sort out things down at the truck and see you both shortly,' said Cam before tramping down the echoing stairs once more.

'So I'm going to give you a little needle in your hand, Danielle, just in case we need to give you some fluid.'

'What's your name again?' Danielle asked.

'I'm Sydney, and that other bloke is Cameron.'

'Sydney, you guys should really just leave me here, seriously. I'm not worth it, don't worry about me, just leave me here—' Her voice began to break.

Syd interrupted. 'Danielle, so, that's not going to happen. I'm sorry … no, I'm not sorry. It's not good that you're upset about life, but I have a job to do, and right now, that is looking after you, giving you this needle, getting you down those damn stairs, and then off to hospital. So, even if I did want to leave you here,' he smiled at her, 'I'd surely get in trouble from *someone*.' He gently tapped her hand, looking for a vein. 'And besides, Cam wouldn't let me leave you here; way too much paperwork.'

Danielle smiled back and looked at Syd with big, wet eyes. 'Thank you Sydney, you're sweet.'

'Ha! Don't be fooled Danielle,' he said, as he continued searching around her plump arms.

'I know it doesn't look like it, Sydney, but I'm *just a normal person*, you know,' said Danielle confidently.

'I'm sure you are Danielle, but I can tell you that *your veins* are not normal,' said Syd, still searching, 'they are so difficult to find.'

'I'm just lonely.'

'That's no good.'

'I don't want to be alone anymore. I don't want to die alone.'

'I don't think anyone really *wants* to die alone do they?'

'Do you think I'm going to die?'

'We're all going to die, Danielle.'

'Today, I mean.'

'I don't think so, but how would I know?'

'You're a paramedic.'

'I can't predict the future though, unfortunately.'

'I know. I'm just lonely. I just don't want to be alone.'

'I know Danielle. How long have you felt like that?'

'Last few years. I lost my job, a couple of times, and later had a really bad break-up.'

'What changed at eleven-thirty tonight? And, please, just hold still, there'll be a little scratch in the back of your hand.'

'I just woke up and felt something was diff— arrgh, ooh that hurt!'

'Just stay still for me, Danielle, I've almost got it, the slippery little ...'

'Okay, okay, I'll try. Arghh aaar—'

'Mmm, Danielle, you moved and it blew the vein. I'm going to have to do another one. You have to stay still for it, okay?'

Cam soon returned and helped Syd spend the next ten minutes finding a vein on Danielle's enormous arms. Cam finally found one and successfully cannulated after Syd's two failed attempts.

The second crew arrived, and it took all the strength of the four paramedics plus another ten minutes to prise Danielle out of her recliner.

Cam was relieved not to find the cat underneath her.

With determined coaching, positive reinforcement, and a good deal of sweating, Danielle was able to stand on her good leg, before flopping into the stair chair and being strapped in.

For the next ten minutes Syd and Cam controlled the top half of the stair chair and the backup crew held the bottom of it. The stair chair; a sturdy metal and plastic chair with wheels and a retractable tread system, allowed the paramedics to move Danielle down the stairs smoothly. Usually, a single operator could manage a patient in it but Danielle required four, and every one of them earned their thirty dollars in that hour.

From arrival to departure, Danielle's job took ninety minutes. The trip back to ED took two.

Two years earlier – Karen

There is nothing as anguished as a mother at her child's funeral – the evolutionary misdeal is as perplexing as it is devastating. As Karen watched her child's coffin being lowered into the ground, she felt an inexplicable sense of failure and defeat. What was the point of anything now?

Jessica, Karen's firstborn, died at a friend's backyard party three weeks ago. The funeral had to be postponed because the autopsy results were initially inconclusive. Eventually, it was concluded that Jessica had collapsed due to hyperthermia and had died from choking on her own vomit. She had reportedly taken one tablet of ecstasy. Another thing that shocked everyone involved - save the investigating police - was that Jessica was found to be six weeks pregnant. Jessica was fourteen years old.

The morning of the funeral was clear. It had been planned for early in the day because the past week had been hot and muggy, and serious state-wide storms were predicted. Although the sky remained clear, there was a hot breeze, tormenting the mourners around the young girl's grave.

Once all the lovely and inconsequential words were spoken, Karen and her husband Jerry stood side-by-side and hugged the friends and family members one by one. Even though both of them thought they had run out of tears long ago, fresh ones flowed. Eleven-year-old Riley clung to her mother's dress, and looked on with an expression of indifference. She knew her sister was dead, and she clearly understood what death was, but the how and the why were beyond her despite her constant questioning of her grieving parents.

She noticed her father shy away from her mother whenever they were alone together. She heard them argue a few days before the funeral and understood that her father blamed her mother for Jessica's death. Karen had let Jessica attend the birthday barbecue that afternoon, which was to have become a supervised party later that night.

Karen was led away to the cars by her aunt while Jerry stayed with Riley, holding her hand. Jerry spoke politely with the minister who conducted the service, keeping Riley firmly by his side. A boy with white-blond hair approached her.

'You're Riley, right?'

She glanced up at her father's back as he spoke to the minister.

'Yep,' she replied.

'Hi mate, I'm Lyndon, I was, well, I am, a really good friend of your sister's.' His face was long but his eyes were definitely dry. 'Here's my number if you ever need anything,' he said, passing her a scrap of paper.

'Like what?' she asked innocently.

'Just someone to chat to, about your life. Your sister's life. Your family. Whatever. I'm here. Your sister was special to me.'

'Okay. Thanks. I think.'

'I gotta go,' he said as Jerry turned to Riley, noticing only Lyndon's lean form as he walked away.

Jerry and Riley headed for the cars to drive to the wake, both of them noticing the cool change, the breeze raising goosebumps on Riley's bare arms.

Karen's tears ceased when the storms came at noon. The river flooded later that day, and parts of the city were evacuated.

01:40 hrs – Princess Alexandra Hospital Emergency Department

Danielle's transfer from ambulance stretcher to hospital bed took nine people. Many hands make light work in most cases; not so in this one.

Cameron's handover was quick and succinct, and Danielle could still not come up with a time, or even a day, when she first felt the left-sided weakness.

Syd rolled the stretcher outside while Cam started on the paperwork.

'Hey there stranger, how are you feeling?' Sonia asked as Syd disinfected the stretcher.

'Hey Sonia, what are you still doing here?'

'I collected my car and went out to another job and now I'm back here, and being in this ambulance bay is just a fun place to be, you know?' Sonia said sarcastically.

'Well here, take some anti-microbial, anti-fungal, hard-core disinfectant and get scrubbing on this feral stretcher,' Syd said. 'Actually, have you got a match?'

'Feral patient?'

'Hmmm, yeah she was … but I felt really quite sorry for her. She was overweight like I'd never seen, and lonely as hell, and said stuff like she doesn't want to die alone. I reckon that's pretty sad to be venting like that to someone you don't know.'

'She was talking to you both about it?'

'Nah just me, Cam was downstairs organising. You should have seen the unit she lived in. It was like the tip. Unbelievable.'

'Was she a hoarder? Mmm, I've been to a few of those. Eye-opening and nostril-closing, that's for sure. And, now you've probably got even more on your mind, eh?' Sonia spoke kindly.

Syd paused. 'I suppose,' he said, as he finished cleaning the stretcher.

'Like I said before, just let me know if you need a hand. With anything.'

'Thank you, Sonia. It means a lot for you to say that. And I will take you up on it once I've given tonight some thought and if it turns out to be difficult. Plus, I may need some advice about my assessments later.'

'No worries at all, Sydney,' Sonia said with her familiar smile and strolled back to the ED.

Syd needed to walk. He set off down the driveway leading to the public hospital car park, narrowly dodging a small pile of loose bricks and gravel on the way, which was barely lit. A large building shadowed the car park, and the few dull streetlights on the far side did little to lighten the gloom. The scattered, scudding clouds were lit faintly from beneath as though the sun was setting.

Sonia poked her head into the write-up room, told Cam she was going to talk with Syd, then walked out onto the street. When he wasn't there she assumed he must've gone to the car park – there were few other options.

At the entrance to the car park, she could see a male figure with a similar build to Syd's approaching her quickly. She thought it might somehow be Syd, since not many people frequented this car park after midnight.

'That was a quick bit of fresh air,' she said lightly.

The figure grunted and Sonia could now see his white-blond hair – it wasn't Syd. She sensed that the man was trouble and wasn't surprised when he thumped her shoulder hard with his as he passed.

A few steps away, she could see Syd standing directly under a light, and called out to him. 'Hey,

Sydney! Did you see that arsehole just then? He barged me as we passed!' She turned but the man had disappeared.

'I thought I saw someone, but he didn't speak to me,' Syd said. 'I thought you were staying up there with Cam. Are you okay? Are you hurt?'

'Yeah, I'm okay, thanks,' she said, rubbing her shoulder. 'I know you probably think everything is fine, but it's so much better to get it off your chest before it causes issues—'

'I know Sonia,' Syd interrupted, 'maybe I'm just not ready to talk yet. I think I said that before.' Syd didn't want to come across like an impatient know-all. He liked Sonia. She was an ICP who kept her head and didn't pull rank.

ICPs, also known as Alphas, were sometimes known to have 'Alpha-tude' – where they mistook their professional standing for personal superiority. Alphas had more drugs to dispense, different tools, and different responsibilities, but were still simply paramedics helping people who were in trouble. Some Alphas were just plain dicks. Then again, so were some Bravos.

The student paramedics, like Syd, were Charlies.

Sonia, Syd had judged, was not one of the 'dick' ICPs. She had been a Bravo paramedic straight out of university and had learnt the essential skill of knowing how to talk to people, a skill not taught at high school or university. She applied for and was promoted to ICP two years after starting, and held the crown as the youngest ICP in the state at twenty-two years of age. Most of her peers respected her for it.

'I know, maybe you're not ready to talk. That's fine. I'm just making sure you're not going to go walkabout.'

Syd gave a gracious smile and thanked Sonia.

'We should probably both be smoking shouldn't we? Standing under a street light in a creepy dark car park?' Sonia said.

Syd chuckled, 'Don't even joke. It's two years since I quit the demon cigarettes and after tonight I—'

'I'm sorry I even mentioned it,' she interrupted, attempting to keep the conversation light. 'Don't take it up again. Smoking is the—'

Sonia's phone lit up in her chest pocket, illuminating her shapely torso and soft face. 'Ah it's comms. We've been talking for too long obviously.' She pressed the glass screen, turned from Syd, and said, 'Hello. Sonia.'

Syd noticed himself smiling before his mind fell back to Amber making love with Sebastian, waking up beside each other and later having breakfast on Southbank, watching the river flow through the city, being playful and close and laughing together. Making memories together.

All of his memories were a lie. *He* was the 'other

man', the 'affair'. She must have enjoyed running the risk of being caught: Syd knew Sebastian lived in the city, and Syd and Amber often went to dinner with friends there or to other social events. He tried to make some sense of it. Maybe it was just that he led the predictable life of an honest and trustworthy shift worker and she took advantage of that? He felt humiliated for telling her he loved her, but he did truly love her. He wanted her forever. And her claim that she felt the same way seemed feeble.

What was wrong with her? Why would she do that? Why say things that weren't true? *Why live a lie?*

He felt loss, deep loss. Again, his mood darkened. Then he remembered the loss he felt in the embrace of Ken's wife earlier this evening. He told himself that he didn't really know loss – Ken's wife, *she* knew loss. The saddest kind.

He thought about the dream he had had at station, and how, even subconsciously, he must want to live 'happily ever after'. He knew himself well, but was still being shown aspects of his life he had not really considered until tonight. His patients were adding to the pressure, and his personal life felt as though he was being pushed into a corner with no chance of repose.

Suddenly Sonia was there before him, eyes wide. 'Cameron's been hurt. Let's get back up to ED.'

Nine years earlier – Danielle

The click of Danielle's high heels turned the heads of the men in the office. Her legs made them linger like schoolboys with one-track minds. Their jaws would drop as she passed, and once she was out of sight, they would catch each other out, and then grin dopily, as if they now knew that perving was a hobby they shared.

The blue woollen dress started just above the knee, contrasting beautifully with her tanned legs, and swelled over her shapely hips, snuggling tight against her waist, then stretching over her full breasts, below a neckline that managed to look attractive as well as professional.

Danielle had the middle of three generously sized

offices reserved for managers, which were separated by walls of glass. She entered her office through a heavy glass door after addressing her secretary and sat at her desk. On either side she could see clearly her two managerial colleagues at their own desks, which looked out and over the floor to their subordinates' cubicles. She had never liked the layout of this office as she often felt closed in. Today, she felt imprisoned. She stood up, and saw the beady-eyed director loitering outside his office, raising a coffee cup to her with a smile.

Her stomach sank and she felt a sudden urge to vomit. Instead, she returned the smile. Danielle had been taught in the early days of working for this company that a weakness shown is a weakness proved.

She picked up her phone and pressed a speed-dial key. 'Rebekah, we need to have a meeting about the merger. Now.' Rebekah soon appeared and coolly strolled past Danielle's secretary and into the office.

Rebekah's professional responsibilities were on par with Danielle's, but she lacked the same ambition.

'Good morning colleague,' Rebekah said after the glass door whispered shut, 'are you okay?'

'Fuck no. Francis the Fucker is all over me now,' Danielle replied. Both the women kept their faces expressionless. They knew they could be seen by their competitors.

'What happened last night? Did you finally give in to him?'

'Absolutely not. I wouldn't let that pig touch me if life on earth depended on it. I went home not long after you.'

'He was trying it on Cindy earlier on in the evening, I heard. And then, what on earth was he thinking mixing his drink with yours and downing it like he was at a uni party? In front of everyone!'

'*How* on earth is he still here?' Danielle asked.

'You know how: by keeping the women he is sexually harassing under control with the promise of promotion. You included. You shouldn't stand for it Danielle. If you don't contact that support group, *I* will, and get his arse fired.'

'I know I should. But then the promotion goes out the window though doesn't it? And senior staff will all think of me as the woman who got the Fucker fired. I'd be an outcast.'

'Why give a hell about the promotion? Look where you are now!' Rebekah caught herself showing too much expression. She glanced left, then right, and then purposefully straightened her face and leant back in the chair.

'I've wanted to be in that role since I started here. It's the only reason I left PWC.'

Women neatly dressed in pastels buzzed about the central open office space carrying papers and coffees as though their minds were paralysed by the ambient lighting.

'I've got the number here,' said Rebekah, sliding a sheet of paper across the desk. '*Again*. Call this later. Not at work. Have a chat. See what your options are. Please. This is no good for you. No good for us.'

'*Us?*'

'Yeah *us*. Women!' Rebekah again had to remind herself to mute her passion.

'Okay, okay. I get it, okay. I'll ring and I'll have a chat.'

'I'm so sick of seeing him drooling over you at work, and then there was that whole turning off the lights debacle. Creepy arsehole.'

'Well, yes, now that was creepy. "I'll turn them back on if you let me touch your hand." Touch my hand? *Really*? He sickens me. Those black, beady eyes. And it's not like I've ever given him a reason to flirt with me.' She looked thoughtfully at her friend. 'I'm *just a normal person*, you know. *And* I just want that job.'

'Ambition is no reason to be harassed. You really should talk to someone about it, someone who can help.'

'Okay, okay. I'll take your advice, I promise. You're the only person I've told about this, you know? But for now, let's call it a day.' Danielle smiled. 'Should we get a coffee?'

'I've had three already this morning. I'm a little jumpy. Maybe I'll just have water,' Rebekah said with a smirk, 'and you really need to talk to other friends about that pig you know. Then tell the fucking world.'

'I don't like telling every*body* every*thing*, I'm just not like that. But I do agree with you about this, I'll contact the support line.'

They left Danielle's office and ambled across the office, chatting openly about yoga. The director sat at his desk and spotted them as they approached his office. He hurried to the glass door to catch them, but the two women had seen him move and increased their pace. They were not quite quick enough. Francis the Fucker popped his head around the open door. 'Good morning ladies. Danielle, can I have a word?'

Rebekah rolled her eyes as Danielle said quietly, 'I'll just be a tick,' before sauntering into the Fucker's office.

Francis was one of the directors of the accounting firm and had been with the company for his entire working life. He knew all of the staff on his floor. And he knew what to look for in his employees – apart from the standard degrees and exceptional grades – it was a somewhat submissive personality.

'So, Danielle,' he said as he closed the door behind her, 'how are you today?'

Danielle nodded and smiled.

Francis circled her at a sensible distance as he went around to his chair. 'Have a seat Danielle,' he said, motioning her to sit across from him, 'I won't keep you long. I've just called you in to chat about the senior manager's positions that have been open for a little while.'

Danielle shifted in her chair. She could feel her face flush.

Francis continued. 'I sat in on the partners meeting yesterday, and aside from the merger being confirmed, there are now three senior manager's positions. Infrastructure, Energy O&G, and the one I know you've got your eye on, Healthcare.'

Danielle felt her pulse bounding. Her composure, though, was absolute. She sat upright with one leg crossed over the other, hands in lap, and chin held high.

'I have been very much interested for some time, Francis. And I continue to believe I can lead the Healthcare division to excellent results. I have proved I can work on diversified projects and can face and manage the complex challenges in this field. I am excited about the future.' Danielle's heart rate settled. She looked directly into his untrustworthy eyes.

'Yes, yes. I do know that. Thank you Danielle.' He pushed back so far on his leather chair that it reclined almost horizontally. 'There's not much that happens in this office, Danielle, that I don't know about.' He squinted at her before jackknifing on the chair and resting both forearms on his desk. 'And that's why, I have been informed to tell you, that you are ...' he paused.

He could hear Danielle's shallow breaths. Her face was pale. She felt her bottom lip break gently from the top. The view before her had dwindled down, from Francis' whole office, to his face, and now to his mouth. The box closed around it with each word he spoke. That is all she saw.

'Unsuccessful. Smith, Stewart, and Waters have been given the jobs. They have been asked to keep it quiet for the next week.'

Danielle felt the words like a punch in the chest. The air was forced out of her. 'I'm ... unsuccessful?'

'So sorry Danielle,' he said smugly, 'but those guys simply put out better numbers than you do, and lead their teams with more, ah, how do I say it ... nous.'

Danielle crumpled in the oversized chair. 'Nous?' She looked at the director. 'But, I've worked much harder, than Smith ... and —'

'It's okay Danielle, you'll still be leading your current team, as small as it is; it's still an important element of the firm.'

Danielle tried to speak but no words came. Her lips quivered as her clear eyes became wet. 'You said I was ... I was a, a shoe-in,' she forced the words out while trying not to sob.

'Well, that was a while ago now, wasn't it. And, frankly, your performance since then has been a little lacklustre.'

'I've put in … all my time, my life,' she said as the tears rolled across a thin layer of foundation.

'And that's a good thing Danielle. You should be proud of that. And I'm sure positions will come up eventually.'

'Eventually? Come on Francis,' Danielle stared at her hands as the teardrops fell into them. 'No. Hold on. Actually, this isn't happening, is it? This is you being funny. This is not a good joke Francis.'

'I'm not joking Danielle,' he said.

'I know you, Francis. You must be joking, right? One minute you're coming on to me, next minute giving me devastating news about my career? Yeah right, I don't—'

'Danielle. Hello? Are you in there? You didn't get the position. And I have no idea what you're talking about – *me* coming onto *you*? It's probably better for you to take the rest of the day off and we will see you tomorrow.' He was as implacable as a brick wall.

'You want me, to go … home?' she said, unconsciously chewing the inside of her cheek.

'I think that's probably a good idea at this stage Danielle, yes.'

'And, I haven't got … I haven't got the promotion?'

'No, you haven't.'

'And, there were three positions, not just two?'

'That's correct Danielle. I'm sorry you didn't make it.'

'And, my performance, of late, has been … has been, a little, lacklustre?' She gripped more inner cheek between her teeth.

'Yes, it has been a little, Danielle, yes. Look, I'm really sorry about it, but you and your team can still improve and you know you are still an important facet of the firm.'

'Yes, you've already said that Francis.' Danielle looked at him through saturated eyes and running mascara. 'Do you remember the time you turned the lights off and came into my office?'

'Innocent mistake, that was. I wasn't sure if you were even still there or not. You know that Danielle,' he said, his voice expressionless.

'And you walked up behind me and touched my hand?' she said softly.

'Well, I was guiding you through a report spreadsheet at the time.'

Abruptly, Danielle launched stood up, slamming both hands down on the desk. She stood over Francis and stared. He continued to sit there, gritting his teeth and widening his unfeeling eyes. 'And what are you going to do about it? Bitch.'

Every muscle in her arms burnt. The iron taste of the blood filled her mouth. Her vision was speckled with black at the edges. Francis' sickeningly strong cologne filled her nostrils. She could feel her breakfast begin to rise in her throat.

He stood up powerfully and glared back at her. Danielle slowly moved her face closer to his and turned her head to the side. If they weren't both snorting air like conquistadores, it would appear they were about to kiss.

Francis broke his stare and quickly looked down at her mouth. As he did, Danielle spat a liberal mouthful of blood-laden saliva directly into one of his eyes which spattered his cheek and ear.

She stepped back and covered her mouth with both hands, eyes still wide and shocked.

He looked across at her with one eye, then wiped the other eye clear of bloody spit. His movements were measured and deliberate, as if he were savouring the moment.

'Oh Danielle,' he said before sitting back and reclining, 'professionally, this is one occasion you are going to regret.'

01:55 hrs – Lyndon

They have seen mum and taken her in. I was seen and cleared. This is taking sooo long. Im bored. What r u doing?

Lyndon drew hard on the remainder of the cigarette and threw the butt in the gutter, thoughtlessly sending it on its way to the ocean. He stared at the full moon and wanted to howl, not as a joke, but as a release. He felt energy inside himself that he could not describe, energy that he thought was strangely fuelled by communicating with Riley.

Mum is up n down again. Dad ignores her. I just don't get it!

and

Mum set another place at the table 2night, no1 sat

there. Wtf? Is she nuts? ☹

were common examples of Riley's text messages to Lyndon.

Each and every message took him back to the evening of Jessica's death two years ago.

Lyndon and Jessica had called each other boyfriend and girlfriend for around three months, and had been having sex for around four months. They had discussed buying some ecstasy tablets to take at an upcoming party at Pete's parents' house, and have their 'sexual experience enhanced' in Pete's bed. They had both been told by friends that it was a great decision, despite neither of them having had sex for very long at all.

Lyndon never had to get parental permission to go anywhere, and he felt a little lost without any boundaries. He drifted, and was cast into the big bad world of drug use and addiction early in his teens. He had been buying weed and pills from an older guy at school, who was sixteen and dressed like a banker, and rightfully so as he was doing well for himself.

The day of the barbecue party was dry and hot, and everybody hung out around the pool for most of the day, swimming, sunbaking, and chatting. Pete's parents were always around and were good supervisors, making sure the twenty-odd teenagers behaved safely, but they didn't shadow them too much or spoil their fun.

When the sun went down, Jessica followed Lyndon into the kitchen where they grabbed a can of soft drink and ran upstairs to Pete's room. They swallowed a little pink pill each. Lyndon told Jessica that the banker had said, 'These pinkies have a higher percentage of MD, so it'll be even better.'

Then they wandered back downstairs, where, within ten minutes, Jessica's condition began to deteriorate.

At first she dismissed the attention her friends were giving her, saying that she must have eaten something that upset her stomach, when in fact she hadn't eaten anything all afternoon. Her good friends gathered around, refilling her glass with water, over and over, watching her guzzle, unable to quench her thirst. Lyndon asked what the matter was, and she said she felt hot and sick. Lyndon thought it was maybe just from having fun in the sun.

In ten minutes Jessica projectile vomited and collapsed on the grass near the pool. Despite there being twenty-five people aged between thirteen and seventeen, plus three adults, nobody checked Jessica's airway or even thought to roll her on her side. Pete's parents immediately called the ambulance.

The closest ambulance crew was delayed. They were three minutes away from the party house but had been sent to a forty-year-old woman who had a toothache.

The ambulance took twenty minutes to arrive. By that time, Jessica was dead.

De shrink just said mum haz to stay. Shes in deep I think. Not bout me I hope? I have to stay here coz Dad aint home. Shitballs!

He needed to get into the hospital. Somehow, Lyndon thought it more sensible to attempt to break in, find his way to the mental health department, and then help Riley, rather than walking through the front door. Most people would think Riley was simply a bored thirteen-year-old girl, but Lyndon thought that it was his responsibility to help her. He hadn't been able to save her sister.

Just the thought of Jessica produced a fire in Lyndon. He had met Riley only the one time, but she messaged him regularly, and told him things that made him feel like her big brother. He thought he advised her wisely. He'd never had to fill this role before and felt he was doing some good now.

Lyndon had also been injecting crystal methamphetamine for the last two months and tonight a rage burnt inside him. The cool air hit his hot face but he didn't notice the temperature. He felt his stomach sway with every message from Riley, his mind never far from her sister. He parked the car and read Riley's last text.

Lyndon's options were limited, perhaps due to circumstance, but more likely due to his innate lack of common sense. Thinking he would make it through to the mental health wing quickly and effortlessly, Lyndon stormed from the car park and up to the ambulance bay. As Cameron swiped his pass to enter back into the ED, Lyndon timed the swing of the brick perfectly.

01:55 hrs – Amber

Amber told the mental health admin desk operator that she was an off-duty ED nurse, looking to pass on a message to Doctor Marcia, who was doing rounds in the psych ward tonight. Amber was then politely told that Doctor Marcia was with a patient right now and could not be disturbed. Amber felt particularly discouraged when, even after producing her hospital identification, she nonetheless had to sit in the small waiting area outside the admin office.

Near the only visible power socket, Riley sat against the wall, with her mobile phone charging while she urgently tapped at it. Amber sat across from her, and for the next five minutes the two sized each other up by exchanging glances. A couple of times their eyes met and they both smiled.

Amber wanted to take her mind off recent events, hence her need to speak with Marcia, and broke the silence with Riley instead. 'How long have you been waiting?' she said. Riley jumped, then smiled and said, 'It feels like forever. Like, I'm not sure what time we got here, but now my mum is in there. She's been in there for, like, two hours.'

Amber raised both eyebrows and uncrossed her legs. 'Are you okay with it?'

Riley took a long breath in, ready to reply in the most unnecessarily comprehensive way possible, before she remembered that she was in the mental health waiting room, and, like, who the hell was this crazy chick anyway?

'Yeah, I'm okay. Thanks.'

Amber grinned, recognising Riley's defensive nature. She could see herself in the girl.

'My mum was a bit erratic when I was young,' she said, 'but it eventually turned out okay.' Riley nodded and forced a smile. 'Hi, I'm Amber. I'm an ED nurse; I'm just waiting for my doctor friend to chat with a patient in there.'

'Hi Amber, maybe your doctor friend is the one figuring out my mum? That'd be a bit crazy, if they both came out at the same time and, like, one walked to you, and, like, my mum walked to me.'

'Oh that wouldn't be too bad, because then all

four of us could go out and have a super early breakfast somewhere nice.' Amber wondered if young Riley would get the joke.

'Ha ha, yeah totes that'd be comfortable wouldn't it?' Riley said, not fully understanding.

'I think it'd be okay after a while, after we all forgot about our jobs and our problems. I'm sure it'd be fine. We're all just people, really.'

'*Just* people? That's a funny thing to say.'

'Well we're all people, you know. We could all go and have breakfast. I don't think it would be a problem.'

'Yeah but, like, you don't know my mum,' Riley said with a warning tone.

'Yep that's true, but trust me, my mother and I had our issues when I was your age.'

'How old do you think I am? And, like, how old are you?' Riley was now facing Amber and had forgotten the phone.

'About fourteen or fifteen? Is that right?'

'I'm fourteen in July. Do you think I look older?'

'Well, we can't speak about age until you tell me your name, you know ...'

'I think I look way too young. So annoying. I'm Riley.'

'Hi Riley. And you shouldn't be worried about looking too young. I think you are very pretty,' Amber said kindly.

'Some of the kids at school who are my age *act*

like they're old. And how old are you? You didn't say.'

'Yeah, it's just human nature isn't it, to always want what we don't have? When we're young we want to be old and appear mature and grown up and to rush in and experience everything like we can't wait, and then, when it's done, we want to reverse it all. It's kinda silly really,' Amber's mind floated away a little before snapping back. 'And I'm twenty-six. I'm happy with my age.' Amber didn't sound too convincing, even to an almost-fourteen-year-old girl.

'*You're* very pretty. I love your hair,' Riley said confidentially.

'Thank you Riley,' Amber said. 'What's your favourite subject at school?'

'Hmmm, I don't really have a favourite. I have to make sure I'm the best at *every* subject.'

'That's a fair bit of pressure to put on yourself.'

There was a long pause before Riley opened up. 'Like, I know right … but it's not, like, me … it's my dad, it's just that I've gotta get good grades for him and it was stressing me out today, that's why I'm here you see because Mum called the ambulance, who brought me in to see someone to talk to, and Mum came with us, but then the people in there said I was fine and they *still* have Mum in there.' She paused again, this time for breath.

'How come your dad isn't here waiting with

you?'

'He's overseas. He's usually travelling somewhere for work. I miss him and I think Mum does too. We have a strange family sometimes. Well, it's been stranger since my sister died.'

'Oh no.' Amber let the words hang. 'You probably have quite a story, Riley. I'm happy to listen, you know, if you need someone to talk to. We all need someone to talk to sometimes. That's why I'm waiting for my doctor friend. I need to talk to her. She knows me—' Amber interrupted her own digression, 'but hey, I'm happy to chat to you.'

Riley moved directly across from Amber and positioned herself comfortably, with only two metres separating their seats.

Amber felt butterflies stir inside her and could see her own face at thirteen in place of Riley's. She forced another smile and noticed herself blinking excessively. She found it difficult to look into Riley's eyes. Riley stared, intrigued to realise she felt instantly comfortable chatting with this woman – a first for Riley.

A full two minutes passed before Riley spoke, which seemed strange to them both. The silence made the time seem longer, but warmer, and the two felt closer.

'I just had a panic attack, that's all it was. Why I was in here.' Riley took a measured breath. 'What I mean is, the ambulance brought me here *because* I had a panic attack, and couldn't control my breathing. I'm not crazy.' She smiled. 'Hopefully my mum isn't crazy either.' Her smile faded.

'And how are you feeling now? After it's all finished?'

'I feel good. I feel fine. But, like, I am actually worried for Mum. I never really think about what is, like, going on with her, 'cause she's, like, my mum.'

'And that was worrying you today?'

'Hmmm, not really … I was worried about what my boyfriend was doing. That's what was worrying me.'

'What was he doing?'

'Just, like, texting me stuff about my sister.' She repositioned her legs. 'Well he's not, like, my full boyfriend. But we chat a lot.'

Amber understood. She nodded, glancing at Riley and each time seeing herself more and more clearly.

'Maybe he'll be good to you. Is that what you think?'

Riley squinted. 'He's already good to me. But, he's not my boyfriend, he's just, like, a friend.'

Amber's expression remained the same, calm and kind. 'You said that your sister died. Why would he text you stuff about her?'

Riley didn't think twice before she replied. 'Because he cared so much for her, and he also cares so much for me. He's, like, a great person, and I know he loved my sister very much.'

'How old is he?'

'Nineteen.'

'Oh,' Amber said as she slid back into her seat. 'And your dad? I know you said you miss him, but is there any chance you could spend more of your time with him when he is home?'

'Yeah, we do. We spend loads of time hanging out when he's home. But, he's away more than he is home. And yeah, I know what you're saying.'

'And he's good to you? Your dad?'

'He is, but he grounds me if I don't do what he says, or, if I don't do what I say I'm going to do. But he's usually very kind to me. He's a happy dad.'

They both smiled slightly.

'He sounds like a good dad. You should cherish him.'

'Except when he stresses me out about school.'

'I suppose he just wants the best for you though, right?'

'I suppose.'

Amber sensed Riley didn't want to speak about her father any longer. She left another long pause before changing the subject.

'So, this nineteen-year-old guy, your not-full-boyfriend, do your parents know about him?'

Riley's comfort evaporated. 'My mum knows of him, but, like, neither of them have met him. He's just a good friend, not my boyfriend. I'm sorry I even said that. And apparently he knew my sister really well. That's, like, what's kept us close.'

'So, he's more like a brother than a boyfriend?' Amber said, noticing her friend Doctor Marcia walk out from a door near the admin desk. They saw each other and Amber pointed a finger, signalling for her to wait and Marcia nodded.

'Oh no,' Riley said hurriedly, 'that's, like, feral. He's not like a brother at all. He's such a great guy. He really cares for me. He says the nicest things. No way, not a brother at all.'

'How often do you meet with him?' Amber spoke gently.

'What do you mean?'

'Do you see him every second day … or once a week … or just whenever?'

'No. That's not it. We've never met up except when I saw him at my sister's funeral. That's, like, the only time. I still feel close to him though.' Riley sounded slightly defeated.

'Okay. That's okay. You're allowed to feel close to him,' Amber leaned forward and put out her hand. Riley gave it an apprehensive look, squeezed her own hands together, took a deep breath, and then placed her hand in Amber's. Marcia coughed in the background as she stood waiting.

'I know you're not asking for my advice,' Amber said, 'but I can really see my younger self in you. Almost down to your eyelashes. I remember when I was almost fourteen and how I didn't like to listen to guidance from anyone, so I don't expect you to take my words seriously. I'd still like to tell you, at least for my own sake. Is that okay?'

Riley nodded.

'I want to tell you so much, and I know everybody's circumstances are different, and I also don't know the full story of your life and the people in it. But,' she paused and took a deep breath, 'firstly, you should love your dad and be as close to him as you can. It sounds like you two are already pretty close and that you have a good relationship, I urge you to hold onto it and to not forget how good that is. And to love your mum too. She may need more love than your dad, but you have to never forget that family is number one.' Amber's eyes began to glisten. 'Secondly, and I know you're not going to like hearing this, but you need to not spend any more energy on the nineteen-year-old guy. When it all boils down, nineteen-year-old guys are really only after one thing, and the direction your life may take if you follow that path will be rocky and unnecessarily difficult.' Amber's eyes filled with tears, and Riley watched in amazement. 'Love will come to you. Let it. Don't rush.'

The speech should have been too much for an almost-fourteen-year-old girl to process, but it wasn't. Riley soaked it up; she sat with wide eyes and an open mind. Still, it didn't make a dint in her attitude. 'And what makes you such an expert?' she said as she let go of Amber's hand. The door tinked shut as Marcia gave up waiting and escaped.

'Riley, honey, I am definitely no expert. At *all*. But I know what I still struggle with in life. And I know why. And I want you to avoid that. Maybe this conversation will help, maybe not. I hope it does.'

Riley grabbed back Amber's hand and nodded.

'We all have faults. Nobody is perfect. I just hope that there are strong seeds of independence growing in your mind. That's what I hope.'

Amber stood up to leave. Riley's grip tightened.

'Good luck, beautiful Riley,' Amber said, then left by the same door as Marcia.

Riley squeezed her fist firmly and placed it to her lips. She pushed up an armrest to allow her to lie down on the chairs.

She visualised her future and what she wanted while she left her phone charging at the wall.

01:58 hrs – Princess Alexandra Hospital Emergency Department

Syd followed Sonia, both of them striding back up to the hospital while he shot questions at her about what had happened and how he thought Cameron was in the write-up room. Sonia remained silent, the questions hung unanswered.

As they approached the ambulance bay, Cameron could be seen lying on his back with a nurse and Doctor Das kneeling beside him.

Sonia knelt next to the doctor and put her hand on Cameron's neck to check for a pulse. 'What happened?' she asked.

Doctor Das' tone was as calm and clear as ever, although this time he spoke rapidly and used expansive gestures.

'We have had one nurse assaulted as well by someone who just stormed into the ED. He was highly combative and security has now detained him. But I've no idea what happened to Cameron.'

Sonia looked over Cameron's head as Syd raced into the hospital to retrieve a bed and scoop to put Cameron on. Cameron's pulse was rapid, and he was breathing with no obvious difficulty, but he was most definitely unconscious.

She formed a fist with her left hand and firmly rubbed her knuckles against his chest.

'Can you open your eyes Cameron?'

His shoulders shrugged inwards towards the sternum rub she gave him and he let out a moan as his eyes flickered.

While Sonia instructed the nurse to go and get a bed and two wardsmen, she inspected the underside of Cameron's head, looking for blood or depressions, then, after finding nothing unusual, supported his head for cervical spine protection. The nurse stood to go but was stopped by Syd who returned wheeling a bed accompanied by two nervously fidgeting wardsmen.

The team soon had the large Scotsman on the bed which the wardies quickly wheeled toward the resuscitation area with Sonia and Syd in tow. Doctor

Das had resus filled with assistants in no time, who took a full set of Cameron's vital signs and continued to assess his neurological status. The doctor phoned through to CT to prioritise Cameron's treatment, and then spoke with the other doctors who were assessing the injured nurse.

She had been punched in the forehead and fallen backward, probably suffering a mild concussion. She would stay in a ward bed for observation after she also had a CT scan.

Sonia and Syd stayed with Cameron as he was wheeled into the CT room to see if he had sustained any damage to his brain.

'I really hope he's okay,' Syd said to Sonia as they both peered through the great glass window that flanked the CT room.

'He's a thick-headed Scot! I'm sure he'll be okay,' Sonia said, knowing full well it was a futile comment.

'This is seriously the single most fucked-up night of my life. Hopefully it's not for Cam,' Syd spoke dully, 'he's been a paramedic for a long time, and seen so many different—' Syd stopped himself, realising his words sounded like a speech at a wake. 'I just ... really hope he'll be okay.'

Sonia's phone rang and she answered while the two of them strolled slowly back to the ED. It was management. Although it had been a tough night, they were down a crew and needed Syd and Sonia to be back on the road as soon as possible. Sonia conveyed this to Syd as they entered the write-up room where Wesley, a managerial officer, was waiting.

Wesley was, like Sonia, an ICP but had been working for the company for much longer. While he somehow maintained his skills as an ICP, he rarely did jobs on-road, and was more comfortable being in the office with the other staff who had had enough of paramedic work. Wesley was the type of person who had put so many years into the job that he was now completely burnt out, angry about it, and simply seeing out his years to maximise his long-service leave. He was heavy-set and had a permanent scowl on his face. The previous year, at forty-five years old, - while on a six day holiday in New York - he thought it a good idea to have one of his whole arms tattooed with Native American patterns and designs. The young, newly graduated paramedics loved fussing about where he got his ink done. Not many people knew that Wesley was actually his surname.

He spoke in a dull mumble. 'Hi. Sorry, but we've gotta get you guys back on-road, there's jobs pending and—'

'Would it be okay if we discussed the events that *just occurred*?' Syd was trying not to be angry, but it was obvious.

'But there's jobs pending,' Wesley muttered

officiously and then turned his back.

'Do you think you could hold the phone for five minutes *Weez-ley*, and let me process what has just happened to my partner?' Syd snapped.

Sonia grasped his elbow to calm him.

'So, as a student, you're refusing the direction?' Wesley asked as though holding out the bait as he spun around with wide, animated eyes.

Syd looked at Sonia and saw her gently shake her head, signalling caution. Syd ignored it.

'I'm just having difficulty with the fact that my partner is pretty much in a fucking coma right now and your biggest worry is getting me back on-road and working your pathetic stats spreadsheet, rather than giving some concern to not only *his* condition but also *my* mental health by maybe *pretending* to give a shit.' Syd advanced and stood less than a hand span from the overweight manager. 'You may have been around lots of humans opened across the chest but *I have not*, and I probably don't need *joke management* hassling me after a night like tonight.'

'So, it's all too much for you? The jobs tonight? And, I heard about the stabbing. But are you refusing a direction? I know you've been having difficulty with the assessments too, Sydney—'

'Not the time, nor the place, Wesley,' Sonia cut in, then spun Syd by the elbow to face her. 'You can go home if you like Syd. It has been a massive night for you. I understand. Just go home and relax. Take the rest of the shift off on sick leave.'

Wesley hissed behind him.

Syd turned his head to one side so Wesley could see one eye glare.

'I'll be okay, Sonia. I just think *management* needs to start treating us with care rather than reckless abandon. This isn't the first time I've seen it in the short time I've been working here,' he said, speaking to Wesley through Sonia.

Syd's eyes met Sonia's. 'So will it be you and me working together? Out of the truck or your Forester?'

'You'll both be in the truck. Sonia can get her drugs out of her car,' Wesley snapped.

Syd turned his head half towards Wesley again and gritted his teeth.

'I'll see you at the truck Sonia,' Syd said and walked out. As he passed the triage desk he asked if there had been any word on Cameron. The triage nurse shook her head, and said she had just got off the phone with Cameron's wife Claire, who would be in directly.

Syd had never met Claire, but felt fond of her after hearing so many life stories from Cameron.

02:30 hrs – Lorraine

The flashing red and blue lights had been gone for around twenty minutes, and the street had returned to its normal tree-lined tranquility. Exactly 355 digital photos had been snapped of Ken and the surrounding area by the police, and the coroner had taken his body to the morgue to be examined.

Heather sat on the water feature, still sobbing. The bustle of the police, their constant careful questions, the speed and accuracy with which the paramedics had moved; it all felt like a lifetime ago to Heather, and yet it all hung in the space around her. Blood drops spattered the tiles between the house and front door.

Lorraine stood up and held her mother's

shoulder. She noticed idly that her blonde bob was still neat. 'Mum, we should try to do something about this house.'

Heather, her face in her hands, said nothing. Her eyes were now void of tears. She could not think of anything sensible to say, and certainly didn't care about the house.

'You know who I think it was?' she glanced up through swollen eyes, 'that fucking Neville Nelson! It's all because of Ken's fucking arsehole politician of a boss!' She began to sob again.

Lorraine turned back to Heather, bent down to her, and stroked her face. 'Come on Mamma, get up.'

Heather gingerly stood. Lorraine supported her with an arm around her slender waist. When the two women were side by side, their shared genes were undeniable. Despite the twenty-five years separating them, their size and shape were almost exactly the same.

They walked up the stairs and onto the porch, peering through the front door. They both stopped and noticed each other in the massive mirror. 'God I hate that mirror,' said Heather, 'except that you're in it. I love that bit.' They both fashioned a smile.

The Cagney and Harlow images looked murky, as though now coloured by the dark puddle of dried blood on the floor nearby. Heather's face was pale, and she felt her stomach starting to lurch.

'No. No. I can't go in there! Not like that!' she cried, but only Lorraine was there to hear her.

'Just come through to your bedroom, Mum, and try to get a couple of hours' sleep. You're exhausted. Frazzled. Just lie down. I'll take care of you,' Lorraine said reassuringly as she led her mother through to the bedroom.

'He was a good man, your father,' Heather spoke softly.

'Ken was not my father, Mamma. I know you're upset, but are you feeling okay?' Lorraine drew the heavy curtains.

'You know what I mean, honey. He was good to you … good to us, for those years.'

'I suppose,' Lorraine said uninterested.

'What do you mean "*suppose*"? You love Ken, I know you do,' Heather started to sound annoyed.

'I know, Mamma,' Lorraine's tone now mimicked her mother's, as she pulled a sarcastic face. 'Anyway, Mamma, the curtains are closed and the doors are shut. No chance of being seen or heard. We can talk now.'

'Okay, honey.' Lorraine slipped off Heather's shoes as she lay down and closed her eyes.

Lorraine looked calmly at her mother. 'I followed Bradley out to Morningside earlier. I knew he was selling to Ken.'

'How did you know that, love?'

'I heard Bradley on the phone months ago

speaking with him. The words he was saying, the details. I just put two and two together. Then I started paying special attention. And I learned that Ken was buying for his boss. You're right, Mamma; it was for that Neville Nelson.'

'I fucking knew it. And because of him—' Heather gulped and sniffed.

Lorraine turned to her mother. 'I don't know if tonight had anything to do with Bradley.'

'I don't know either, honey. I'm just upset.' Heather's eyes scattered around. 'Jesus Christ, why didn't you tell me he was buying drugs for that politician dog?'

'I wasn't one hundred per cent sure about any of it until tonight. They were both very careful, so I studied and prepared, but I only saw the deal tonight by fluke, I promise Mamma.'

'So it *was* that Bradley then?'

'I'm not sure Mamma. But don't you worry about him. He'll be getting his soon enough. Next time he shoots up.' Both women now spoke in a clear, placid whisper. Heather sat up, red eyed but enthusiastic, 'So you switched it?'

'Yep. But only his personal supply. Bradley, that piece of shit; the man is truly an idiot, but I could never work out where he stored the clients' stock. I would've loved to have been able to get the right stuff into that politician's veins.' She leant forward to her mother's ear. 'I miss Dad, Mamma.'

Heather smiled. 'Me too baby.' The two women shared a reminiscent stare. 'He's why we're doing this.'

'I want them *all* to get what they deserve.' Heather's eyes creased maliciously. 'One at a time, honey. One at a time.'

02:55 hrs – Alpha 989

'Does this mean you want me to drive?' Sonia's normally perky voice sounded a little broken.

'Yeah, I don't mind doing patient care,' Syd replied, 'if I make it through tonight, I will have ticked off a few predicted and inevitable stressful work situations.'

'Hmm ... okay,' Sonia said as she climbed into the driver's seat of the ambulance. 'Hey, have you seen the city at night?'

'Not yet, but I'm pretty tired —'

'Well, let's go for a quick drive to the river. It's really pretty, and there won't be anybody hanging around tempting us with their luscious-smelling barbecues or picnic lunches.'

'Ah, okay then. Are we allowed to just drive there?'

'Already covered. I told Wesley that we needed to talk about tonight. It's all about the student's positive mental health you see,' she said speeding off.

'Why is that guy such an arsehole, seriously?'

'Wesley? He's always been like that to students. He thinks he knows everything. He's been in the job for too long.' Sonia drove quickly. 'And it's as though he lives in a state of constant depression. In fact, that's exactly where he is.'

'Well, that's no reason for everybody else to have to deal with it. Get some help. He's a bully, and not only to me.' Syd paused as the shops whizzed by. 'Fuck him. Fuck his depression. After Cam got hurt tonight, he didn't give a damn, just couldn't wait to swing his dick around to make us get back on-road. He didn't even ask how Cam was.'

'I know you don't like him, but it's probably better for you to play nice. He is one of the senior assessors at the SDU, you do understand that right?' She looked over at Syd. 'He could make your life very difficult.'

Syd chose to keep quiet for a while, his body loose and lurching around with the bumps in the road as Sonia zipped the ambulance towards the river.

After a few minutes of silence, Syd said, 'Yeah. Maybe. Still. Fuck him. Karma will look after Wesley. I don't know what's going to look after Cam though, but I hope it's something good.'

'I hope so too,' Sonia said. 'So! Onto bigger and brighter things. How long have you been here in Brisbane?'

'I moved here from New South for the job about nine months ago.'

'What did you do before ambulance?'

'I was a jackaroo and station hand then did a bit of travelling, and then got this job. Is this like another job interview?'

'A country boy, hey? So, you *used* to make food for people, and *now* you're saving people's lives, oh, you melt my heart,' Sonia said cheerily as she drove on autopilot. Syd smirked at her, but was unsure how to take her comment.

'Um, well, thanks, I suppose. And *I* know your story, well, everyone does really. You are quite the record breaker and child genius I believe?'

The ambulance arrived at Kangaroo Point, a cliff top by the Brisbane River that offered an amazing view. Over the other side, the city was alive with bright lights and made for a spectacular skyline.

Sonia parked, taking up two spots; there were no other cars or people around.

'Well, I definitely am not a child genius, I can tell you that for sure,' she said, hopping out and walking around to the river-view point as Syd did the same, 'and I can also say that nobody knows my story, well, not the full story anyway. I've made a point of it. Too many gossips in this business.'

'That sounds a bit lonely,' said Syd, leaning onto the stone wall and looking over the city.

Sonia turned to him and inhaled deeply. 'Yeah, maybe it is,' she said.

'So, what's the full story?' asked Syd. 'Where did you come from?'

'Well, one day, my mum met my dad, and fell very, *very* much in love, and, later, when they had been in love for the appropriate length of time and—'

Syd shot raised eyebrows and a grin her way. 'You're joking right?'

'Of course I'm joking. I'm being hilarious and getting away from answering the question,' she grinned. 'You don't want to know too much, Sydney.'

'Good one. You *are* hilarious,' Syd said sarcastically, paused, then spoke out to the river in a different tone. 'And you don't have to tell me, that's okay, but I would like to know.'

Now Sonia paused and considered, then said, 'So, pretty much, I never had a place that I would call home until I came back to Australia and was fostered at fifteen, over in Perth to start with.'

'How come no location until fifteen? Did you

know your folks?'

'Yeah, I did. We travelled the world spreading the word of *the lord our saviour,*' Sonia waved both hands mockingly. 'Well, *I* didn't, but my parents did. I couldn't actually get into it. *Ever,* really. My parents didn't mind though. I never spouted on about how I thought differently than they did, even when I finally fully understood my feelings. They were okay with me just keeping busy. I think that's probably what kept my head in the right place after they died.'

Syd turned to Sonia silently. She was already looking at him, her face half lit by the orange of the street lights and the other half by the moon's white light. The city glow on her blonde hair, shining, gleaming, was brilliant and bewitching. Her eyes were clear, and he could see little full moons in them when she faced him.

'So, I came to Brisbane after Perth, with an aunt and uncle actually, who had been estranged from my mum and dad before their death. They had always liked me and they really looked after me. Quite amazing people. I love them both very much.'

Syd and Sonia stood about a metre apart, looking towards the city. No people were walking the street, and they could hear no cars, only the river gently lapping, one hundred metres away from the top of the cliff on which they stood.

A quiet city of two million. No unruly sounds.

The faint scent of Sonia's perfume and a background of pretty city lights. Syd forgot his fatigue and felt energy surround them. The night's suffering and stress drained away.

'So, yeah, I suppose, that's where I came from,' said Sonia.

'Well you do have a reputation for being a child genius, just so you know, because of the whole *youngest ICP in history* thing.' Syd changed the subject.

'You hardly need to be a genius to run this gig,' she said, smirking, 'and I just get bored easily, that's why I applied for it.'

'*I* can't even get through the beginning of the ACP Diploma! How stupid do I feel?' Syd said.

'Hold on, I thought we were talking about *my* life,' said Sonia.

Syd raised his eyebrows and waited for her to laugh, which she did.

'Yep, well, back to me,' he said, 'now I'm stupid *and* selfish.'

'You are definitely not stupid, Sydney. You don't actually think you are, do you?'

'No, I don't. At all. But I've never had a self-confidence issue until I started at SDU. The teachers made me feel pretty useless because I failed some initial exams in the start-up program. It really threw me. It was as though they actually *wanted* me to quit. Cam has been helping me a lot with it all. He's a legend. I really hope he's doing okay.'

'I'm pretty sure he'll be alright, I've got a good sense for these things.'

'I hope so, he's a good human.'

'Sure is.'

'So, what else do you do besides hold the youngest ICP title? Anything fun?'

'Well, okay, so it's my interview now is it? I read a lot. Lots of fiction. I have about six books on the go right now. I have three dogs who I run every day, rain, hail or shine—'

'Is that their names?'

'Wha'? No. I run them, no matter the weather. Derr!'

Syd pretended to recline on a sofa, put his hand on his chin and said in a calming voice, '*Hmm, now how does that make you feel, Sydney?*' then replied, 'Well I started to feel very, very, extremely, life-changingly stupid after I had a conversation with a colleague named Sonia.'

They both laughed.

'That *is* a pretty good name for three dogs though! C'mon!' he said.

'Yeah I suppose it's okay if you're a weather nerd,' said Sonia, still beaming.

'Do you play any sports? You keep pretty fit.'

'Only the work team's Oztag when I'm not working. And thanks.' They both fell silent for the next minute, the two of them comfortable with each other.

'I've always wondered why they don't turn all those lights off through the night. Those buildings over there are offices, not apartments. Surely nobody is working *right now* – well, maybe the cleaners are – but not in —'

Syd began to point and count aloud each illuminated office window. 'I dunno, *that* many offices anyway. What do you think?'

'Easy; it's so the rarely seen night-flying, black-tip-winged southern red goose doesn't fly into them.' Sonia said. 'Common sense really.'

Syd laughed. 'Where do you come up with this stuff?'

'I've got a good imagination,' she said. The silence returned. 'And what do *you* do for fun, Mister Worthington?'

Syd took a long look at Sonia, and smiled before answering. 'Well, aside from trying to study and understand the systems involved for doing this job well, I have also gone skydiving but that's been on the backburner since I've moved up here. Oh, and I would normally play touch footy but I haven't found a team yet.'

'How many jumps have you got?'

Syd chuckled. 'That's a funny question, particularly when skydivers ask it.'

'Why is it funny?'

'Because some really good jumpers have low

jump numbers and some poor jumpers have really high numbers. It's not always about the number, it's more about how current you are, kind of.'

'Oh. So, how many jumps have you got?'

'Not many. And I'm not current right now at all. But I do love it.'

'Great. So, how many jumps have you got?'

'Maybe 350-odd.'

'You don't know the exact number?'

'No, and that's over the last five years too. I've lost my log book and got new gear, and blah blah blah ...'

'So, 350-ish times you've jumped, of your own accord, from a non-crashing plane, and have not been attached to someone else who was in charge of the parachute?'

'Yes. Wow. I'm glad we've sorted that out and you finally understand.'

'Smart arse. But that is pretty cool. I really respect that, because I don't think I could do it alone.'

'Different strokes.'

'I have done a tandem though.'

'And loved it?'

'Of course! It was really exciting. I just don't think I'd want to be in charge of all that.' She said pointing above her.

'That's surprising,' Syd said as she looked over at him, 'because you're always so in control with work, and you direct people well.'

'Thanks. I don't know if I've given it all that much thought really.'

'And that's okay, you know,' Syd said kindly.

'Hmm, maybe, I am intrigued though. Just to overcome that fear. I don't like to be scared of things. I'm of the opinion that as soon as I recognise a fear, I'll do—'

'As much of it as possible to get over it?' Syd interrupted as Sonia nodded. 'Yes, me too, I am of that exact same mindset.'

'It's a good mindset to have,' Sonia said, then jokingly changed tack. 'But, I could've said *that I'll do everything in my power to avoid it!*' She laughed. 'Is that what started you skydiving?'

'I don't think so.'

Syd noticed Sonia smirk. 'Truly. I always just wanted to do it. Just the thought of falling through the sky and safely landing on the ground … I thought it would be so exciting and it was. And *so much fun*. I'm so glad I started it.' Syd grinned. 'But, I used to be scared of needles, so, to get over that, I donated blood as regularly as possible. That worked, I got over it; and now I'm the one jabbing people left right and centre!'

Sonia gave him her cheeky grin.

He took a step back. 'But I don't think I actually know *real fear*. I don't know real chaos. I have led a pretty protected existence so far. Private schools. Good family. Country living. Little bit of travel. It's not as though I've ever had to protect my family from pirates on the Caribbean seas who are threatening to kill my mother and skin me alive, you know? I suppose it's all relative, but when I think about it I feel like a spoilt little shit really.'

'Because you don't know *real* fear and haven't experienced *real* chaos?' Sonia's eyes looked huge.

'Yeah,' Syd replied.

'Because you were born into a different life to other people throughout the world?'

'Yeah.'

'Well, I don't think you should feel guilty about that. Nothing you can do about it. Actually … maybe, just be a good human.' She grinned at him. 'And I reckon you're doing a pretty good job of that.'

Ten years earlier – Lyndon

The supple pillow smelt sweetly of fabric softener. The room was neat; his toys were all either packed up or proudly displayed. The bedroom window was open, and overlooked a vast sugarcane field from the second floor. A gentle breeze blew intermittently and caught his pale hair. But he didn't stir.

The moon looked close and colossal, and if he were awake he would lie and stare out at it in amazement, wishing he could touch it.

The house was old, by Australian standards, and almost every step an adult took produced loud creaks and squeaks which echoed through the rooms.

He lay, sleeping peacefully on his side, as a child does who is safe from harm at three in the morning.

Suddenly, the erratic flapping of large wings sounded just outside the window, followed by a growl and a single bark from a dog further away.

Lyndon didn't stir. Each breath he took was perfect, quietly in and out, as if he slept in a bubble of contentment.

After a while, there was a stretched and spacious noise, a wooden groan like an ancient tree resonating as it was about to crash to the earth, a sound that came from only one spot in the house when an adult's weight was transferred to it. Inside Lyndon's bedroom door.

His eyes flickered open then shut. It was the smell that woke him. Sickly sweet rum. He dared not move, hoping that he was having a nightmare, and safety would soon greet him with the morning sunshine.

He had been in this nightmare before.

It hurt every time.

The rum smell came closer and he soon felt a strong calloused hand stroking his hair. The calloused hand undid his nightshirt and held his chest before pushing him onto his back.

Next he felt the tiny pricks of rasping wood against his face. It wasn't pushed hard against him, and it didn't hurt, but he knew exactly what it was: a three-sided mask of a female face from the front and each side. At the top of each face, the face of a white woman, was a feminine gold patterned headdress pointing down the forehead to furiously shaped eyebrows. Each facet of the face shared an element with one another – each blue-shadowed eye served two facets of the one face, as did each of the blushed cheeks. The mouth of the front face stopped at the top lip – there was no lower jaw – as though the mouth was wide open.

The adult-sized mask covered Lyndon's tiny face, aside from his lower lip. He had seen it on another occasion and the three-faced image was burnt white-hot into his nightmares. Much like the one he was in now.

The rum mouth, surrounded by sparse wiry beard hair, pushed down hard onto the bottom half of Lyndon's face, slobbering repulsively on his mouth and chin. Lyndon winced and cried and struggled for almost thirty minutes while he was assaulted and raped, dreaming only of escape, to fly and to drift away.

Later he heard the floor creak again as the rapist left the room with the mask in hand.

***

His white-blond hair was again shifting in the slight draught, this time from a different window, the breeze less on this side of the house but the light stronger. He stood about a metre away from a queen-sized bed, looking over the rapist.

Every part of him ached, the type of ache a child should never feel, an ache that started at the end of his light hair and went through to the core of his bones.

Tears fell from his eyes. He didn't sob though. He was void of emotion after weeping for the last two hours. He was drained of energy, and any hint of love was sapped from his heart.

The sun's first ray entered the room and touched Lyndon's cheek. His tears evaporated and he felt oddly and immediately safe, before accidentally dropping the cane knife he had held with both hands. The long wooden handle thudded hard on the floor and the thin blade clinked so loud that he thought the house might collapse. Lyndon's eyes widened and jaw dropped and lungs held in his breath as he froze and saw the rapist sway his head, then rub his face, then turn onto his side facing Lyndon. The rapist's eyes remained closed and he seemed to return to sleep.

Lyndon bent down to pick up the knife, its length half his height. As he did, the rapist's bed partner turned over and sat up, saw Lyndon, then said stridently, 'What do you think you're doing in here?'

Without further thought, Lyndon picked up the cane knife with one hand, stepped up to the bed and with one ferocious two-handed swing, planted the blade into the temple of the rapist, cracking the skull, wedging it behind one eye and close to the bridge of the nose.

Vivid red blood squirted as the rapist screamed and clutched and spasmed. Before long, dark blood pooled while the rapist began to seize, then flounder, and eventually die.

Later, Lyndon was moved to a new foster home.

04:30 hrs – Alpha 989

Sonia and Syd had been given a job while they travelled back to the station. The crew that had helped with Danielle needed more hands and strength with another job they were on. Despite the two crews working together as quickly as they could while still using safe lifting practices, it took the four paramedics an hour to get the obese male patient out of his house. The other crew continued with their treatment and Sonia and Syd returned to their station.

'I can't believe we made it back. What happened to *'a heap of jobs pending'* Wesley? Dickface,' Syd said, leaping out of the truck and striding through the station's plant room.

'I'm going to make a cup of tea. Would you like something?' Sonia asked after taking a quick look around the station to get her bearings.

'No thanks. I'm going to lie down.'

As soon as his head hit the pillow, Syd relaxed. He sank into the stiff, single bed as though a cloud enveloped him. He dreamt of the sky and the freedom when he jumped, as though he could break away from everything on the ground. He escaped the thoughts of Amber kissing Sebastian, and Cameron's unknown and worrying condition. He pushed away the memory of Ken's wife, and the desperation in her grip, her need. He relinquished the thought of the house-fire patient with the skin peeling from his face.

Syd felt as though he were flying, head down, feeling the breeze against his body, and listening to the constant grey noise of the oncoming wind.

As he flipped himself from head down to a sitting position, he felt a tug at his jumpsuit, and saw Sonia, mid-air, undoing his fly.

All of a sudden, he awoke with a gasp and saw Sonia standing in the light of the half-opened door to the bedroom in which he slept.

Confused and a little panicked, he said, 'Oh wow, I thought we were skydiving together,' and then sat up to look at her.

She said nothing, and let the door shut quietly behind her as she stepped closer. The darkness was sudden, as were Sonia's lips on Syd's.

'Sonia?' he said. 'What are you doing? Are you okay? Are you sleep-walking?'

'I'm fine Sydney. I know you've been thinking about this,' she said in a pensive tone, 'I know.'

Syd could think of nothing to say, but thought yet again that tonight was the strangest night of his life.

She unclicked his belt and as she began to undo the clip of his pants, she felt the vibration of her pager. She had a quick look at the blue illuminated words then handed it to Syd. 'We have to go. Come on, Sydney.'

Syd barely had time to agree before the door slammed open to a blinding yellow light and the silhouette of Amber standing there like a Roman soldier.

'What the fuck do you think you're doing?' she screamed. Her face was red with anger. 'You have to get up! Sydney!' Amber's nasty voice slowly morphed into Sonia's kind tones, 'Sydney!'

'Sydney?'

Syd's eyes opened to a vibration on his hip, a bright light, and the view of Sonia standing in the open doorway of his room with her pager in hand. 'Come on. Get up. We might have a sick one,' she said gently.

Syd sat up, realised what had happened, and then clumsily zipped up his boots.

05:35 hrs – 43 Ferguson Skyline Drive, Seven Hills

Syd hardly noticed the weight of the heavy oxygen pack, as his thoughts were focused on the job in front of him. Ted gave Syd and Sonia his wife's medical history in two vague and questionable sentences while he led them the short distance through the house. Sonia asked Ted if Audrey had any cardiac history, to which he replied politely that she most certainly had, she had had a heart attack less than a month ago.

He went on to explain how the paramedics had been remarkable, and how he was confident that the same level of professionalism would be repeated tonight.

When asked where Audrey's medications were, Ted explained that they were scattered around the house; although he seemed unsure of what they were.

He presented Syd and Sonia to Audrey.

Audrey sat bolt upright on a dining-room chair which leant against the kitchen bench. Her eyes were wide with fear, she was dripping with sweat, and her face was blue. When she attempted to speak it sounded as though she was drowning.

And she essentially *was*.

Syd held her wrist and felt a rapid radial pulse. He dropped the ridiculous oxygen kit, unpacked the CPAP mask, handed it to Sonia, and wrapped the elastic harness behind her head to which she attached the mask. The oxygen mask would ensure the continuous positive pressure of oxygen in her lungs.

Sonia assessed blood pressure and heart rate, which were both predictably high. She had opened her drug kit on the nearby kitchen table and set a small bottle of Nitrate, an Aspirin and all the goods for cannulation.

In sync, Sonia asked the husband, Ted, and Syd asked the patient, Audrey, if she had any allergies. Ted replied with an unambiguous 'No'. Audrey continued to sound as though she was underwater but Syd thought he caught an aqueous negative.

Sonia handed the Nitrate to Syd. He then put

both his hands into Audrey's hands and told her to squeeze them, which she did. He checked for other contraindications to the medication by shining his torch into both her eyes to check for equal pupil reaction. He then asked Audrey to lift her tongue to the roof of her mouth, before lifting up the oxygen mask and spraying the Nitrate below her dry tongue.

'Is she going to be all right?' Ted asked softly, sitting close behind the crew. 'It was all just so sudden. We went to bed and everything was fine, then she wakes me up and says she feels heavy in the chest again. So I brought her out here to get a drink of water.'

Sonia handed Syd the foiled Aspirin and slid the cannula kit towards him. 'We're just going to do a few tests on your wife first, okay Ted? We've already started treating her, and I think we may be on the right track. But I'll tell you in five minutes or so, okay?' She briskly walked the few steps to the kitchen sink and poured a half glass of water, handing it to Syd.

'It's our sixtieth wedding anniversary next week. She keeps telling me so I won't forget,' Ted said in the background. 'How could I ever forget sixty years with this wonderful lady?'

Audrey was attempting to chew up and swallow the messy Aspirin, half of which dribbled from her mouth. Syd gave her a small drink of water, and then had to pry the glass from her desperate hands.

Sonia attached ten plastic stickers to Audrey's torso and to the left side of her chest to assess her ECG.

'Wow! Sixty years. Ted, you must know each other pretty well after that amount of time. You should be very proud,' she said with characteristic sincerity.

Syd had explained to Audrey he was about to put a needle into her arm and asked her to try to keep still. She was an obedient patient. She was in trouble and she knew it. As Syd cannulated Audrey, he wondered what a terrifying feeling it would be to have basic breathing taken away. Essentially, that is what was happening to Audrey, probably because of heart failure; the flow-on effect was that her lungs would fill up with fluid, especially at this time of the morning. Starting from the bottom of the lungs up – drowning from the inside.

Syd remembered the reason he quit smoking two years ago and took a deep breath.

'I don't know what I'd do without her,' said Ted.

Syd thought of the first moment when babies are born and take that first deep breath and into a loud, ear-cracking cry, working new lungs to move air in and out. And in and out.

Nobody thinks about it, of course. How often through life would anyone ever think about it? How grateful would someone be for the breath they just inhaled?

Generally people would be fine until they 'ran out of breath' from running or exercising, or maybe something environmental like inhaling smoke, making them huff and puff. But actually having *the very first thing they were ever given* taken away from them would be so alarming, it was almost inconceivable.

Syd secured the cannula with a wrapping bandage. The sticking plaster would never hold with Audrey still sweating liberally.

'Is it five minutes yet?' Sonia asked.

'Four,' Syd replied.

Audrey's face still had a deep shade of blue, but they noticed a pinkish tinge pushing through.

Aah! Perfusion! Syd thought, before he checked Audrey's vital signs, and then lifted the oxygen mask again to give her another Nitrate spray.

'C'mon Auds, love, don't you get too sick now love. We've got some real partying to do next week,' Ted said, supporting his wife, trying to look calm but obviously and understandably stressed.

'Just you relax sir. Your wife is in good hands,' said Sonia while she read the ECG. 'So you said Audrey had a heart attack? Was she told she has left ventricular failure maybe?'

Ted shifted in his seat. 'Oh I don't remember what they said. Yes. Maybe. Maybe not. Maybe something like that?' Ted spoke with the sincerity of a man who loved his wife like no other but simply had difficulty remembering medical terms.

'I know it's difficult, Ted, but this time if the doctors tell you what to do, you'll have to do it. It may save Audrey's life one day,' Sonia said kindly, then spotted a bottle of GTN on the other side of the kitchen. 'I can see that little red bottle of Nitrate there on the counter. Did you give her any of that before calling us?'

'No. I don't even know what that's for,' Ted replied, bowing his head.

'Ted, it's okay. It's not a problem,' Sonia's upbeat tone returned, 'this time it's okay.'

'She's going to be alright?' Ted sat up, hopeful.

'I think so. Tonight, she may be alright. But you guys have to know each other's medical needs a bit better, okay?' Sonia's eyes creased as she smiled sweetly. She spoke as if she were speaking to her grandfather, or someone whom she loved very much.

Sonia tried calling comms three times on her hand-held radio, which was predictably unsuccessful. She stayed inside the house, close to Syd, and rang comms from her phone instead, giving them a SITREP of the job so far.

Syd spoke to Audrey continuously, giving encouraging words with every positive change he saw. After another ten minutes, her colour returned, she ceased sweating, and her eyes grew calmer. Her breathing had improved but she still gurgled with each breath, and he told her not to try to speak.

Sonia went back to the ambulance to retrieve the stretcher. Ted left his seat immediately and slowly returned to Audrey, bringing a chair with him. He sat next to her and held her hand. Syd noticed the elderly hands of the two of them, the bony frailty encased in translucent, paper-thin skin.

Their hands melded into each other, as though paired that way from their beginning. Syd lost concentration, transfixed by such a simple thing, something he felt was important – a connection between two people, fused by love. It was something that could never be faked, or copied, or lied about. It was something that would never need to be a status update. It was theirs and theirs alone.

The many lines around Audrey's eyes wrinkled as she smiled.

'He's always had such cool hands,' she said.

Syd jumped back to reality and said, 'Ah, that's lovely Audrey, but remember no talking for the time being okay? It just makes your breathing work harder.'

'Cool hands, warm heart,' Ted said with a grin. 'You know what, love? Don't speak, just take it easy, like the Commodores' song, "I'm easy – easy like Sundee mornin', mmm yeah eee aah..." I'm sorry son, what's your name?'

'That's a great song Ted. Have you ever thought

of a singing career?' Syd said lightly, making them both smile. 'I'm Sydney by the way, pleasure to meet you sir.'

'Ah Sydney, what a name! What a place!' Ted gently let go of Audrey's hand, gave her a smile and went to the nearby bedroom, returning with a framed black and white picture. He took his wife's hand, melding once more, and then said to her, 'Love! It's Sydney!' Then to Syd, 'That's where we met, back in 1956! I remember it like it was yesterday.'

Syd thought maybe Ted's memory wasn't what it used to be until he saw the picture Ted was holding, with the Sydney Harbour Bridge in the background.

'See, this was our engagement party twelve months later,' Ted presented the picture proudly.

They sat at an indoor table which overlooked the harbour. Ted looked strong in his smart suit with a serious look on his face and a good hairline which had been ruthlessly Brylcreemed and neatly combed in the style typical of that era. Audrey looked striking with a glowing cheeky smile, hair pulled back taut in a neat ponytail wearing a dress which hugged her nicely shaped arms, an oversized collar, and a knee-length explosion of tightly ironed pleats. Their hands were together in the photo, just as they were now.

'What a great picture. You don't see that anymore,' said Syd.

'Well of course you don't, that was the fifties!' Ted chuckled.

Syd smiled, 'You don't see *that connection* much anymore.'

Audrey sat between the two men, calm but still wearing the oxygen mask. The hissing sound of it filled the silences. Sydney paid close attention to Audrey.

'I'm sure you *do* see it, and it *is* out there, surely. It just may not be obvious to you Sydney,' Ted spoke helpfully. 'Sydney. Sydney. I do like saying that, Sydney. Great name. Great town.'

'I wasn't talking about *me* in particular—'

'I can see it Sydney. You're a good bloke with a big heart. Eventually, she'll show up.'

Syd scrunched up his face. 'Yeah, I thought she had shown up until earlier tonight—' and then he remembered he was supposed to be caring for Audrey, rather than pouring out his 'big heart' to her husband. 'But thank you, Ted. I think you love your wife very much. It's sweet to see.'

Audrey had settled, and butted in, saying through the oxygen mask, 'Oh Ted, just leave him alone,' in a caring grandmotherly way. Syd opened his eyes at her as if to say *'Don't speak'*. Audrey took the hint and, being the good patient she was, followed orders and remained silent from then on.

Her state had greatly improved and Syd continued to monitor and treat her accordingly.

Soon she was loaded onto the stretcher and into the ambulance. Ted came with them, riding in the front and chatting to Sonia for most of the twelve-minute trip into hospital.

Audrey's condition remained stable throughout. At hospital, she was assessed and reviewed the same as anyone who presented with a recent cardiac history and current acute pulmonary oedema. Ted and Audrey were further advised on her medical condition and would hopefully both be better prepared for the next time if this morning's events were repeated.

Syd felt he understood what Ted and Audrey had together – the absolute love – and thought it fundamental to what he wanted in life. Surely it would be impossible to have that with Amber, a woman who was deceitful from the beginning. From the first time he asked her out, she had lied about everything. Could the connection that Ted and Audrey had be forged in the same situation he and Amber were in? His mind dizzied again when he thought of the relationship he had held so dear. One minute he wanted to forgive and forget, the next he never wanted to see her again.

Twenty years earlier – Amber

Her eyes opened sharply as her little lungs inhaled the single gasp that woke her. The front door slammed, then reopened harshly and she heard her mother yelling profanities for a solid thirty seconds, before there was the sound of spinning wheels.

The door closed gently.

She lay on her side and stared at the glow-worm bedside light and listened for the familiar sound of her mother's desperate cry. It was not long coming.

Amber rolled back her bed covers and rubbed her eyes. Most children her age would stay in bed, make some kind of noise, and await a parent.

Amber didn't have that option. She was an only child to a mother who strove for the dramatic and who insisted on having those around her appreciate the troubles in her life. And, as much as Amber's mother loved her, Amber always came second to her mother's own priorities. Amber knew that she was the one who would comfort her mother.

Her mother would expect Amber to be her helper and caretaker well into Amber's teens, but would simultaneously dismiss her unexpectedly.

Her mother would often ask if Amber was hungry and despite her answering no, would still place food in front of her. While shopping, she would ask if Amber liked a certain dress, and even though Amber would reply politely 'no', her mother would still give it to her for a Christmas gift.

Her self-involved mother forced Amber to act as *her* mother from an early age.

Tonight, Amber's tiny printed socks muffled her steps as she padded towards the bedroom door. She peeked through, trying to avoid being seen or heard at all.

Through the slit of the open door, she could see her mother, sitting on the floor at the top of the staircase, leaning against the wall. Her wet, vividly red hair dangled through her hands as she held them against her face.

Amber could hear her whimpering. She gently opened the door and looked around, then ran over to her mother.

'Are you okay, Mummy?'

Her mother gave a startled jump as Amber hugged her, and then curled her up into her arms with obvious love. She tried to force herself to stop blubbering.

'I'm okay, baby. Mummy's okay. Daddy's just gone for a quick drive, that's all,' she lied.

06:30 hrs – Princess Alexandra Hospital Emergency Department

The ED was now full of natural light, making it look much older and somehow less sterile. The bright LED lighting was always on but only made a difference to the darker corners during daylight hours. Morning had broken, and with it came new crews for each shift.

Audrey had been transferred to a bed in resus. She was now stable and speaking full sentences with no gurgles or drowning sounds, the colour in her face returned to normal. It would not be long before she was reassessed and most likely taken to a ward bed for observation before returning home, hopefully with a management plan. Ted sat patiently in the room designed for waiting.

Sebastian lay in a ward bed, soon to go home. He had had surgery through the morning hours and the surgeon was confident there would be few complications with his recovery as long as Sebastian followed instructions. Sebastian remained completely oblivious to events between his girlfriend and his paramedic. He had thought Sydney's behaviour strange when he last saw him and told Amber about it, once she returned an hour later it all was forgotten. She told him that paramedics had to move quickly at any given minute to make certain they got to jobs *'muy rapido'*. He respected Sydney for his commitment, and then laughed at Amber speaking Spanish. She stood with her hands on her hips and her lips pursed. Sebastian happily kept eating chocolate before falling asleep. They didn't speak of Sydney again.

Bradley was moved to the Intensive Care Unit, near the ED. He remained heavily sedated, with a tube down his throat to sustain his breathing. Airway burns were a worrisome possibility. The burns to his face were of medium partial thickness and healing times were not possible to predict. The burns would be reviewed regularly and an appropriate treatment plan put in place over the following two to three days. He had no next of kin on record, and nobody had come to see him. There were, however, two detectives assigned to wait nearby to interview him when he woke up.

Danielle's left-sided weakness remained throughout the nurse's and doctor's assessments. She then had a head CT scan which uncovered a small blockage to the blood flow on the right side of her brain. Due to the unknown time she had been showing her stroke-like symptoms, her treatment options were limited. The left-sided weakness would most likely persist and arrangements would be made by the hospital staff of Subsidies and Support for her to be rehoused and cared for.

Riley remained in the waiting room of the Mental Health facility, napping occasionally on the comfortable seats, otherwise sitting like a cocoon staring deeply into her mobile phone screen and tapping away with both thumbs as if her life depended on it. She continued to text Lyndon and, despite receiving no replies, she texted with a different mindset, one she felt was more mature and independent. Her mother, Karen, continued being assessed by a senior psychiatrist to 'work a few things out'.

Karen's assessment turned out to be much more thorough, and necessary, than Riley's. The counsellor there had given her a new medication script and advice on dealing with her depression. The lead psychiatrist at the hospital was called in and did a comprehensive assessment of Karen's mental state, dealing with states of change, depression, bipolar disorder as well as suicidal tendencies. One of Brisbane's leading private psychologists was contacted, who had ties to the public system, to further assess and treat Karen. This private psychologist had also recently appeared in the local newspaper, having been awarded the state's highest decoration for mental health support. It was a page three colour spread of him shaking hands and smiling with the Minister for Health, the Honourable Neville Nelson.

Lyndon's strength was surprising given his body size, and yet he had injured Cameron, a triage nurse, and two security staff. He was finally handcuffed and then sedated in ED, and would be assessed by the mental health team at some stage that day. Most of the ED staff witnesses assumed he had taken some form of methamphetamine. When the sedation wore off, he thought of Jessica, and his lingering sorrow returned.

Cameron sat upright in his ward bed with his wife Claire nearby. He had been cleared of any bleeding on the brain, and was diagnosed with a mild concussion. He was soon to be released and he would return home with his wife. Wesley had interviewed Cameron and filled out the relevant paperwork and would be reporting and crawling to senior members of management once they arrived at work.

'How are you feeling now?' asked Syd.

'Ah, bit of a bump,' Cam replied rubbing his head with one hand and holding Claire's hand with the other, 'but I'll be all right.'

'Does he seem any different to you Claire?'

'Aye Sydney, that he does. It's like he's a new man. I've never heard him this quiet,' she said, smiling.

She then said something to Cameron that made them both chuckle, before he gave her a quick, petulant look.

'Was that a private message in Glaswegian that only you were supposed to understand? Because I didn't get a word of it,' said Syd.

'Aye, son. And private it'll stay,' said Cam with a wink.

Syd flicked through Cam's chart. 'Well, I've just ticked you off for a thorough rectal exam in case you injured anything abdominal in the fall, and I think Jeff is on this morning so that's good for you. I hear he has nice, soft, but extremely large hands and a fantastic eye for detail. So enjoy that Cameron,' Syd said as he pretended to sign it and slotted it back into the bed-end.

'Aye, ha, thanks son, that'd be great,' Cam said, ignoring Syd's joke. 'Have you heard who the bloke is that knocked me down?'

'One of the Drug Dependence Unit nurses said

he's a regular over at the needle exchange and that he hasn't been in a good way recently.'

'Yeah? No shite,' said Cam casually.

'She said that he said he actually thought he was breaking into the hospital and knew where to get "all the drugs". Can you believe that? Jeez that pisses me off! Shoots some ice, thinks he's on another planet and hurts several innocent people in the meantime. I hope he goes to jail.'

'Well, mate, he probably won't, but I know what you're sayin'. Me gettin' knocked out is pretty rare thing to happen to ambos here. But people sportin' addictions and hurtin' other people one way or another is pretty bloody common. Don't stress too much about it son. It won't change.'

'Oh you're so wise, Mister Bloody Negative,' said Claire.

'It *won't* change,' Cam repeated, as though reinforcing the reason he was injured. Syd took two steps backward against the ward curtain and saw the raised leg-cast of Sebastian in the bed next door.

Syd clenched his jaw. 'I agree Cam.'

'Oh you're so wise too, Sydney,' Claire said with added sarcasm as if it hadn't been noticed the first time.

'Son, why are you still here? Go home, man. It's been a big night, go back to the station and safely home. Have a good rest. You've got my number. Gimme a call whenever you want all right? We'll have a beer,' said Cam.

'Okay then, I'm out of here. I'm glad you're okay Cam, I really am. Enjoy the rectal exam. Chat later. And lovely to finally meet you, Claire.'

Both the Scots smiled.

'Safe travels, Sydney.'

07:00 hrs – Charlie 989

'Charlie 989, returning to station, out of service. Thank you for your night, 989.' Her voice was chirpy as a morning sparrow, as if rubbing it in that she had just arisen from a peaceful, full night's rest, and he had not. Syd didn't confirm the message, like a grumpy child, and he certainly didn't want to chirp into the emptiness of the handpiece.

The ambulance moved easily along the main road, as most of the traffic was heading the opposite way into the city to start work. Syd thought that even though the night had been possibly the most eye-opening and heart-breaking night of his life, that at least he didn't lead a nine-to-five life. However suited it was to so many people worldwide, Syd did not feel it suited him. He relished not knowing what was going to happen during a shift, the people he would meet, and the sights he would see. To help people on a day that could be the worst of their lives, knowing that for some it might turn out to be the best. He loved *not* knowing what lay ahead. He thrived on the mystery. And it all came back to the feeling he had chased when he first went skydiving.

Sitting in an ergonomically designed cubicle staring at a computer screen and answering a phone while colleagues talked about their amazing weekend just out of town and TGI Fridays was not Syd's idea of work. Nor life. Nor a good work–life balance.

But, as he liked to say, different strokes for different folks.

He returned to the station, restocked the ambulance and left the vehicle clean. The morning crew were already out on another job, along with the station's officer in charge. The station felt empty and he felt quite solitary. His eyes were heavy and they wanted nothing more than to simply close.

Because he was a student, with no responsibility for signing in and out of drugs, Syd had nothing left to do so he locked up and left the station.

He drove his car down the main road where he and Cameron, and then he and Sonia, had driven through the night. The road was two lanes each way, separated by a wide nature strip, with a speed limit of eighty kilometres per hour. It was now jammed with the nine-to-fivers. The cars and small trucks all drove ridiculously close to one another, all keen to start their 'hump day'.

Syd drove carefully and usually too fast, but at the moment, all the vehicles were travelling at the same speed, as though all joined by a giant cosmic elastic band, which rarely allowed overtaking. Syd allowed a generous space between his car and the car in front. Annoyingly, a blue Audi thought it would get to its destination more quickly, and cut in and filled the space.

Syd sighed, scowled, and held both hands open on the top of the steering wheel.

'Why, dickface, why?' he said in a monotone.

The radio hosts told their jokes and their artificial laughter sounded in sync. Syd backed off the accelerator and recreated the generous and sensible space in front. The traffic on the opposite side going towards the city was regularly at a standstill, and the sunshine heated up early.

The phone rang; it was Amber. Syd paused. Usually, it would be a quick push of the button on the hands free kit and Syd would enjoy being able to multitask, speaking to the love of his life while driving, but now, he doubted the man that the past night's experiences had made him. His choices had been poor. He knew it, and because of this, he questioned himself. The confusion of last night and this morning hung above him like a threatening storm. He had seen Claire faced with the injury of Cam and their closeness afterwards. Syd respected it very much. He had been witness to the actual loss of Ken, and how his wife had to bear seeing her partner dying in front of her. He had felt the love and loyalty in the simple hand clasp of Ted and Audrey and in the way they spoke with each other in a worrying time. He had sympathised with Danielle and the isolation that it seemed she chose to live with.

He wanted to be connected. Maybe what Amber offered was what he needed. He questioned himself further.

Life is too short.

He pushed the button.

'Hello,' he said clearly.

'Hello Sydney, how are you? Was the rest of your night okay?' Amber had a babyish tone.

'No, not really. It was a big night on all accounts. Jobs at work and my life, which you'll bear witness to.' Syd drove even more carefully now he was focused on conversing with the woman who had just broken his heart.

'Sydney, I need to apologise for everything. I'm really, *really* sorry. I don't know what I was thinking.'

Syd waited and thought.

'And it's taken you the four months we've been together to work that out?' he asked with increasing volume and intensity, 'And only because I accidentally suspected it when I saw you walking out of the Argentinian's cubicle?' *The whole four months,* he thought. He tried to relax into the seat, and drove on with the other westward-bound commuters.

'Well, that's what I want to talk to you about, Sydney. I really don't know what I was thinking. It was as if I was living like a rock star, spending time with these two guys ... one who loved me more than anything and showed it more than he said it ... that's you Sydney, it's obvious to me now.'

'So, now that it's obvious to you, you think you may want it?'

'I *know* I want it Sydney. I want *you*. In fact, come over to my place so we can talk face to face rather than on the phone. I really would love to see your face, Sydney.' Amber's tone softened. 'Come over, I'll make breakfast.'

He paused again, thinking hard. 'Last night a few things became apparent to me Amber, and one of the big ones was that I don't want to be alone. I want to be with someone who I connect with, someone I love and who loves me back, who I can share the good and the bad parts of life with, and who'll be with me through it.'

'I *can* commit you know Sydney,' Amber said as

Syd's traffic slowed for a red light.

'You *can* commit? Well that's great that you have that ability.'

'And I *will* commit, Sydney. To you. And you only. That is what I want. I promise.' There was a whine in her tone now. 'You really should come here for breakfast. I'd love to make you breakfast. And, well, you know, we could fool around. I promise I'll make it up to you,' she said.

Syd could hear her gently clacking her tongue on the roof of her mouth. The traffic started again and quickly changed to the regular crawl.

'So, you're offering to feed and fool around with me to make up for what you've done?' Syd said. He knew Amber would sense his wording was aggressive. 'Something sexy?' he added soothingly.

'Well, we've always had that part pretty well worked out haven't we? I thought we could learn something new. Together.'

'That's a bit vague.'

'We can discover something when you get here.'

'So you want us to be together?'

'I know now that's what I want Sydney.'

'And what about the Argentinian?'

'I have already told him we are not seeing each other anymore.'

'What reason did you give him?'

Cogs.

'I told him I loved someone else,' she said. 'I love

you, Sydney.' The traffic continued. Syd watched the road.

'Did you tell him you've been sleeping with me for the last four months?'

'Well, I … didn't say … those exact words, but, more or less … yes, that's kind of what I told him. And that I love *you*, Sydney.'

'And how did he take that Amber?'

'Oh I don't want you to worry about him, or that situation Sydney, just come over for breakfa—'

'You know what, Amber?' Syd said kindly. 'The person I thought you were, was the woman I wanted forever. Maybe I jumped the gun, maybe four months is way too soon to be thinking that far into the future, and forever was definitely way too far, I can see that now. So that mistake was mine alone. Forever though, is not un—'

'Oh Sydney, just stop. Don't be like that, baby, just come over for breakfa—'

'Forever *is* what I want. And the person I discovered you to be this morning is a person I could never trust, and one who I could never love. What you have done is so backward and … hurtful and … deceptive, that I would never be able to have confidence in anything you say or do. I have no idea what part of having another relationship you are addicted to, whether it's the love, or the attention, or the … sex … or that maybe I just wasn't everything you wanted. But I know this … that forever is not what I want with you.' He paused. She was silent, and Syd sensed no cogs grinding away. 'So, from now on, when we see each other at hospital … we will be professional, but that is all. No smiles, no "oh how was your weekend?" bullshit, and definitely no getting back together. And when we hang up from this call, delete my number and never message or call me again.' Syd paused again, choosing his words carefully. 'Things will work out for you Amber. I know that. *You* know that. You control things so they do. I don't know why or how, but it's how you live. And, now, I want absolutely nothing to do with you. Do you understand?' A long silence followed. 'I would like you to answer.' Another long silence.

'Yes,' Amber said quietly, then her voice sounded like it had grown horns and a tail, 'I understand.'

Syd hung up. Another weight lifted from his shoulders. He felt miserable, but free.

Soon after, the mood lifted and he smiled to himself.

The traffic still hadn't eased but Syd thought that the sky looked as though it had grown bigger, or maybe his world had just expanded. One hundred metres further up the road, Syd saw the flash of a dog running across the road on the opposite side. He lost sight of it somewhere in the central nature strip. Syd held his breath and started to decelerate. He couldn't see the dog amongst the bushes.

Suddenly, in a flash of four legs, the dog ran out in front of the car in front of Syd's, the blue Audi. The driver didn't see the dog and hit it at full speed, dragging the brown dog underneath and out past the back like exhaust. Syd had slowed then stopped before coming to the dog, which lay still on the road. The truck behind Syd stopped and the driver got out at the same time as he did to inspect the wounded animal. The traffic in the other lane had slowed but didn't stop. The blue Audi did the same and was quickly lost to sight.

The brown staffy-cross lay still, whimpering, with one obvious broken back leg and massive gravel rash down its whole back, and substantial chunks of fur and skin missing around its neck and head. The truck driver approached the dog with his hand out until Syd told him to wait.

Syd had been around dogs all his life and knew some injured animals could lash out despite the human's best intentions. He walked around the dog and asked the truck driver to get a blanket out of Syd's car while he Googled nearby vets and called the closest one.

Syd couldn't do a full assessment of the dog, particularly as he wasn't a vet, but he spoke with the female on the phone and gave her the best details he could. The vet was happy to receive the dog.

The truck driver told Syd that they could lift the dog together in the blanket and put him on the truck floor for transport. They did so carefully, all the while trying to keep the dog as calm as possible. The dog allowed itself to be handled and never tried to bite either of the men. It looked up at Syd with big sad brown eyes. Syd thanked the truck driver, and followed him the three kilometres up the road to the vet.

Syd and the truck driver carried the brown dog through the sliding doors of the vets, as if they were both paramedics arriving at hospital with a patient on a stretcher. They were met by a pleasant redheaded vet in her mid-twenties, and two younger women, possibly students. The three of them walked through the surgery door and held it open for the men and dog to pass through. They gently laid the dog on the table and took a step back before the women worked fast, assessing the dog's injuries. One of the students grabbed the microchip scanner and read out the owner's address, which was on the road where the dog was hit. She then wheeled a screen connected to a triangular shaped probe with a tightly wound cable.

The vet, whom had given her name as Kate, rolled the gelled probe over the brown dog's chest and a sizable black mass could clearly be seen on the screen.

'That's blood,' she said. The three women all looked at each other with a frown.

'Is there any good trying to fix him, do you

think?' asked Syd.

Kate looked over the dog.

'You said everyone was going eighty? That's a big force. Even though he's stockier than many dogs, that energy has to transfer somewhere. And, unfortunately, it was transferred into this guy's chest.' She squeezed her lips together. 'We'll phone the owners and tell them. We'll make him comfortable. I'll suggest putting him to sleep. I think that'll be best.'

Syd stepped back over to the dog, and looked into the brown eyes of the dying dog, then reached forward and rubbed behind his ear.

Syd's voice quivered and broke as he burst into a quick bout of tears. 'Poor bloody dog.' Kate put her hand on his shoulder and said, 'It's okay, these things happen.'

Syd sniffed, trying to stop the tears, but couldn't. 'It's just an innocent dog. He doesn't know,' he blubbered.

Aside from Kate, the three other people in the room were noticeably uncomfortable seeing someone so upset. Syd sniffed again, wiped his face with his arm and said, 'Big night.'

'Have you been up *all night*?' One of the young students asked with way too much excitement in her voice.

'Yep. More or less. But I am going home now.' Syd took another swipe with the other arm. 'Thank you ladies. I would've been lost if you couldn't have taken him.'

'No problems. Have you got someone to talk to?' asked Kate. 'It's important. But I'm sure you know that.'

Eight years earlier – Sydney

The ute's V8 engine rumbled and slowed just a little as the bitumen road finished and was replaced with graded white-yellow dirt. Large plumes of dust billowed behind the metallic blue tailgate.

They were surrounded by the quality farming land of Victoria. Behind them was the tilted Grampians range, and in front were rolling fields knee-high with wheat, all edged by thick green grass. The cabin of the ute smelt of cigarette smoke and sounded like country music.

Sydney drove with one hand on the wheel, easy and comfortable while his passenger and girlfriend Zarni, gripped her seat with both hands.

'Jesus, do you think you could slow down?' she said skittishly. Syd immediately took his foot off the accelerator.

'Sorry. I'm not driving to scare you. I'll slow down,' he replied.

'It's different driving fast on dirt,' she said, satisfied with his reaction.

'I am driving safely though. I don't want to scare you babe.'

'Well, I'd prefer to finish this trip on a high, Sydney, not wrapped around a tree you know.'

'I get it,' said Syd. They drove on, comfortably and safely, for the next seventy kilometres after which they turned off at a letterbox marked *Agapanthus* onto a smaller dirt road. 'This is it,' Syd said as he drove slowly in past a dirt tennis court encircled by stunning gardens kept in perfect condition. Beds of roses, delphiniums, iris, hydrangeas, foxgloves, were bordered by expanses of velvet lawn where no one ever stepped or sat. The single-storey red brick house was bordered by a wide verandah with two huge chimneys, four immense front windows open to the breeze, and five wide steps leading to the front door. It was a property that looked as though – in its heyday – it would have been a magnificent sight. Now, though, despite the carefully-tended gardens, the house was shabby and worn.

The great front door swung open and a thin, bald

man with a moustache stood there with his arms outstretched, clad in a mustard-coloured shirt and red shorts. Syd pulled the handbrake on and looked at his father. Knowing his voice could not be heard he said, 'Jeez he looks sick.'

Zarni ducked her head to look past Syd out through the window.

'So, Zarni, that's Michael, my dad,' he said.

Three hours later, after the polite introductions and the usual chitchat, five people sat down to enjoy pre-dinner drinks. Michael's wife, Paula, buzzed about and fussed over everyone; Paula's father, Vincent, the original owner and grazier, sat calmly with a half-smile on his face, cut off from conversation by his increasing deafness. The dining room was the showpiece with the most exquisite furnishings; cedar everywhere, in perfect condition and polished to a warm gleam, all of it from the mid to late 1800s. To Syd every single chair looked as if it had been made to be as uncomfortable as possible. There was also a double-ended settee upholstered in black, white and red stripes which looked strange and out of place but when Syd sat on it he realised how comfortable it was. That was until his father started to brag about its value.

Paula soon served dinner – a perfectly cooked traditional lamb roast – which was hailed by all the diners, except Michael. When he wasn't purposefully ignoring his wife, he spoke disparagingly to her.

'Would you *please* fetch me another bourbon, daaarling.'

'I'm almost out of cigarettes. Grab us another packet from the pantry, daaarling.'

'Sydney looks like he wants another, Paula daaarling, grab him a fresh one.'

The man was disrespectful and rude, and Syd was ashamed of his father. Paula forced a smile and bore the treatment for as long as she could before she began shooting dark looks at her husband. He ignored them and continued to speak to her as if she were a servant.

Syd cringed at each word that left his father's mouth. He felt humiliated for his stepmother, livid at his father, and apprehensive about how his girlfriend would regard his father's behaviour. He felt miserable for Vincent, who had grown up on this property, and appeared to be unaware of what was happening to his family despite it taking place directly in front of him.

Then, at one point in the meal, when Michael had left the table and Paula was speaking to Zarni, Vincent leant over to Sydney and whispered, 'Lack of respect is his problem.'

Sydney looked deeply into Vincent's eyes and saw almost ninety years of life's lessons, hard work, and graciousness. He leant back towards the elder and said, 'And he doesn't know how good he's got it.'

Vincent gave a slightly lop-sided grin and nodded.

Michael included Syd and Zarni in the after-dinner conversation, and although it was enjoyable, Syd felt weary of the company. Whenever Paula spoke, Michael immediately dismissed her opinion, tacking on the sarcastic 'daaarling' that seemed to punctuate all of his remarks to her. Paula refused to be ignored or embarrassed, adding her own 'daaarling' to her responses.

It was as though they were at war with each other, and 'daaarling' was their safe word, a reminder that they were married, and should try to get along. If so, it wasn't working.

Michael continued to disparage both Paula and Vincent until Syd and Zarni excused themselves, saying the long day's driving had exhausted them and they needed some rest. Hugs and kisses were exchanged before everybody retired for the evening.

Some time later, while Syd and Zarni were snuggling, Zarni asked abruptly, 'Do you think you'll be like your dad when you're older?'

Syd was taken aback. He didn't know what to say. He was embarrassed by his father and wished he hadn't brought Zarni here to meet him. Syd stared into the dark of the high-ceilinged old room and felt cool air on his chest and face. He searched for the right words. 'Zarni,' he began, 'I haven't seen my father for many years. Actually, this is the first time I've seen him since I've been an adult … And his behaviour is, jeez, I don't even know what his behaviour is … But I'm sorry you had to see it.'

'But he's your dad,' Zarni said.

'Well, yes, I know that. But I *was* raised by my mum. I hardly know this guy compared to her.'

'Hmm, maybe. But you are his blood.'

'Yes, thanks, well I know that too, obviously. It doesn't mean I'm going to be an arsehole like he is though does it?'

'I just don't want to ever be treated like Paula. I feel so sorry for her. She's so smart and lovely.'

'She is great. But, I can't apologise for Michael. It's *his* behaviour, not mine, he's not the same person I am. I can just be embarrassed.'

They heard a heavy thud outside their room, but they both assumed it was someone going to bed who had perhaps had one red wine too many and both quickly dismissed it.

'Do you think we'll live in a house like this? On a farm? Farmer boy?' Zarni's mood changed quite quickly.

Syd chuckled. 'Well we won't know for a little while yet honey. You gotta get through uni still and I've gotta work out what farmin' I wanna do!' Syd's accent was a standing joke between them about the country folk he loved. Syd touched her face and said in his normal voice, 'I know that I want you though. And that I won't ever treat you like my father treats his wife.'

Suddenly, they heard Paula's loud panicked voice from outside their room. 'Get up, get up! Michael! Do something!'

Syd sprang out of bed, threw on a pair of boxer shorts and opened the tall bedroom door to the long wide central hallway. At one end, between the front door and the front room, lay Vincent. He looked so flat it was as though his body had sunk into the floor, with one arm extended and the other pushed up hard against the door to his room. He wasn't moving.

Paula was on her knees beside him holding his face, her eyes wide and appalled.

Michael stood in the doorway of the bedroom opposite, hyperventilating.

Paula was also hyperventilating.

Everyone seemed to be hyperventilating.

Except Vincent.

Sydney rushed to Paula and Vincent then said, 'What happened? What did he do?'

'I just heard a noise, and when I came out he was on the ground here,' Paula said, stroking her father's face desperately. 'Wake up, Dad, wake up,' she said before turning back to her husband, 'Michael! Do something!'

Michael was frozen.

'Okay, okay, hold on, just hold on,' Syd said as he took a deep breath. He gently guided Paula to one side as he knelt by the old man's chest. 'We have to check response … so, there's no response,' he said as if ticking off a mental checklist. 'Now check C for circulation.' Paula had one hand each side of Vincent's face and had pressed her forehead to his. Syd brushed one of her hands away and replaced it with his own, digging deeply and clumsily to find a carotid pulse.

'No pulse,' Syd said. 'I'm going to do CPR now, Paula. I want you to look into his mouth and see if you can see anything in his airway.'

Syd positioned himself with his shoulders directly over the middle of Vincent's chest, straightened both arms, joined both flat hands, and then forced as much energy as he could through to Vincent's heart to push blood around his body and to his brain. Vincent was a burly man, with a sturdy chest, and it required all of Syd's strength to do effective CPR.

Paula fumbled at Vincent's mouth, attempting to open it and look inside, but failed dismally. Zarni, hurriedly dressed in her pyjamas, suddenly appeared beside Paula. 'We just learnt our first aid. I know what to do,' she said. Paula moved out of the doorway and stood behind Zarni as she confidently opened Vincent's mouth, saw nothing obstructing his airway, and told Syd to stop compressions. She then took a deep hurried breath, placed her mouth over Vincent's, and blew hard into him. His chest rose up and then quickly deflated.

'Okay, airway is clear, compressions again,' she said.

Syd continued.

'Paula, is there a phone in there in Vincent's room?'

'Yes, right here,' Paula answered from behind the action.

'Call the ambulance now.'

'It's almost eighty kilometres away. In town.'

'It doesn't matter; we need them to come to us as soon as possible.'

They heard the beeping buttons of the phone as Paula tapped in 000.

'Michael,' said Zarni. 'Michael!' she yelled. It was as though he had turned to stone.

'Dad! Wake the fuck up!' said Sydney in a tone Zarni couldn't contest. Michael shook his head as though he'd been woken from a nap, but he moved slowly and uncertainly.

'Michael,' Zarni said again, 'you and Syd are going to have to alternate. These compressions are going to keep Vincent alive, but it's going to be very tiring, so you need to swap, okay?'

'I've never done this be—' Michael's docile words were cut off by Syd.

'Here, watch me do it. Just copy me exactly.'

For the next forty-five minutes, the four of them worked together with one simple goal: to keep Vincent alive.

The ambulance finally arrived, to the relief of them all. After five minutes of questions and sorting out machines, one of the paramedics told the team that Vincent was gone, but that they had done a great job to try for as long as they did.

Vincent was eighty-eight years old. He had never taken a sick day in his life. Sure, the occasional cough or runny nose, but that would never deter him from living his salt-of-the-earth life and tending to whatever needed to be done on the farm.

And now, he was dead.

Paula crumbled.

Michael froze, then left quickly to wander and chain-smoke.

Syd and Zarni looked at each other as their eyes filled with tears.

Sydney hasn't spoken to Michael since Vincent's funeral.

Zarni broke up with Syd shortly after they arrived back in New South Wales. But watching her manage Vincent's demise sowed a seed deep in Syd's mind, one that remained dormant for years.

08:45 hrs – Sydney

Syd had returned to his car and ignored the two missed calls from Amber and another one from a private number. He sat behind the steering wheel staring at the edge of the knee-high concrete wall, barely visible in front of the bumper. He sat in a trance-like state while a smartly dressed woman delivered her ginger cat in a carry-cage to the vet. He saw her but didn't really notice her. His eyes stung sharply, his mind raced but he felt numb. He switched the air conditioning to full and felt the sweat dry on his face. He shook his head as a wakeup call before putting the car into reverse.

Within an instant, he thought about Danielle and her sadness. He imagined her wanting to escape and thought that the care he had shown her made no real difference to her life. He didn't know Danielle's story, but remembered her desperation as she said, 'I'm just a normal person.' He wondered what had happened to her to make her feel she needed to justify herself. He knew he had judged her, not only her appearance but also her living standards, considering them to be unacceptable and disgusting. He reminded himself that he didn't know her story. What had happened to her. Why she lived that way. Who she had in her life before she became so desperately lonely. He knew, behind every crazy circumstance, there was a reason, an excuse, and sometimes that excuse could lead to a purpose, which some people need to keep on going. Syd thought that Danielle unfortunately lacked this purpose, which might have been the reason why she was in the condition she was in. Syd understood that Danielle felt so alone and scared of dying that way; he felt sadder just thinking there was nothing he could do to help any more. Aside from the damage that was already done to Danielle, from which she might never recover, the only person who could help her any further was herself.

Only she could help herself. Well, *could have* helped herself.

In his mind, an image of her face mixed with a photo Syd had taken while ballooning in

Cappadocia.

The sun's rays formed six strong points in the bluest sky above a blanket of fluffy white clouds. A long, jagged mountain range poked through and pointed towards a single hot-air balloon. Syd loved this picture, this memory, which still brought him solace. It took him away to such a beautiful place.

When he saw the brilliant blue sky, he wanted to escape, to jump, and to travel with his love, Amber. He relaxed as he breathed in the crisp, fresh air. He remembered Audrey's smiling, wrinkled face and the complete love he had witnessed between her and Ted. He imagined what they had gone through together over the last sixty years. He tried to imagine their lives together, what they were like alone, what they were like before they even knew each other. What had made them the people they were? Syd thought of how different life would have been when Ted and Audrey were his age, but got a little lost, seeing as he didn't really know what the dating practices had been back in those days. He settled with the thought of them both picnicking near the Sydney Harbour Bridge, like in the picture Ted presented to him. They looked happy. How did they meet? And, why did they choose to spend their lives together? Maybe they *learnt* to love each other. Maybe they didn't always have the level of respect they have now. Syd wondered deeply if maybe Amber and he could be the same.

He felt at peace as he recalled the floating balloon, and wondered if Ken might now have peace. He couldn't comprehend what Ken's wife Heather must be feeling, and could still feel the anxiety in her embrace. He had not experienced sadness like she had last night – losing someone who had made the ultimate commitment, the lifelong vow of marriage. To have and to hold. For better, for worse, for richer, for poorer, sickness, health, to love and to cherish, without condition, with honour, my best friend, you will not walk alone, I will support you. I will grow old with you.

I do.

And to be stripped of that commitment by someone else, Syd thought, was terribly unfair. But, again he remembered, he didn't know the full story.

He grew even sadder at the thought of his patient's life lessons.

Syd knew the last fourteen hours had affected him, and was trying to be conscious of the effects to his perspective.

His left leg began to shake and brought him back to reality. He put the car in neutral and let the clutch out.

He tried to think of Amber with compassion and consideration. *Why* did she lie? What more did she want from him? Who was she? *Truly*? How did she expect him to forgive her and go back to the way things were?

Each question bounced around an image of Amber. Soon, one of Sebastian emerged, with his olive skin and toothy grin, and lastly his open leg fracture.

Syd had had enough.

Life is too short.

He picked up his phone, searched his contacts, dialled, and sensed a soothing contentment as he listened to the dial tone of Sonia's number.

Jayne. From the beginnings of my ideas for this book, you were an optimistic driving force, and one I could not have started it without. Your ceaseless encouragement, outrageous humour and wonderful love will never be forgotten. Amongst so many other thanks I owe you; thank you for saving me and staying with me in Arequipa. I think about you often, and wish you the happiness you deserve.

Natascha. My first reader and editor, and who initially showed me the way. I thank you for your advice, loaning me books, and for taking care of my dog so many times.

Anna. You understood my passion for this book and your energy towards it was very much appreciated. Thank you for dancing with me. And for Western Australia.

Bronnie. The Kiwi bibliophile adventuring around the world! Your help regarding the overuse of adjectives and producing too-longer-sentences was imperative … I hope! Thank you Bron, especially for the poem.

Gav. To my friend and beta reader; thanks buddy, for your comprehensive report and truthful thoughts. I am seriously lucky to have a mate with so much time on his hands. And who is crazy enough to let me speak at his wedding.

Rosie and Natasha. Two English English teachers touring Africa? Who better to help make sense of my words, delete my long sentences as well as play cards with while we bump around dirt roads that seemed never-ending in a truck that felt as though it had no suspension? Thank you ladies, for the corrections, as well as the laughs.

Vicki. I don't really know where to start regarding the gratitude I owe you. So I'll simply say thank you and I love you.

I have many people to thank for several aspects of this book. Starting at each characters creation through to the production of an actual paperback book, I am lucky to have had the opportunities throughout my life so far for these ideas to have shown themselves to me, in one way or another.

My sincere thanks go out to the many paramedics I have worked with, particularly those of whom that work with a constructive approach, and from whom I have learned how to deal with jobs and how to help the people who actually need our assistance.

Professionally, we all have our own stories, our own experiences, and, of course, our own tragedies. All of which is unavoidably twisted together through our personal lives.

Sometimes we think it is all just too much, and sometimes it is.

Just because we are branded mentally bulletproof most certainly does not make it so.

Everybody, at some stage, needs to talk to someone.

Don't ignore it.

My thanks to John and Todd, and especially the peer support paramedics who truly put their heart into helping their colleagues. You should all be proud of the work you do.

Take care.

Garth Wade was born and raised in Canberra, and attended boarding school in country New South Wales, before working for a publishing company in Sydney. He then left the city and rode a horse nearly every day while working for two large cattle and sheep stations throughout Australia. After travelling around South and Central America, his heart was set on becoming a paramedic, and in 2010, that's what he did, and has been trying to culture the craft ever since. He has enjoyed writing since he was a boy, and now says it is *almost* therapy.

calm to chaos is his first book.

www.garthwade.com.au

www.ingramcontent.com/pod-product-compliance
Lightning Source LLC
Chambersburg PA
CBHW031226120726
47905CB00002B/485